Cutting Remarks

For Mary

Dick Abbott

Re

Cutting Remarks

*Insights and Recollections
of a Surgeon*

*

Sidney M. Schwab,
MD, FACS

Frog, Ltd.
Berkeley, California

Published by Frog, Ltd.
Frog, Ltd. books are distributed
by North Atlantic Books
P.O. Box 12327
Berkeley, California 94712

Cover and text design by Brad Greene
Printed in the United States of America
Distributed to the book trade by
Publishers Group West

North Atlantic Books' publications are available through most bookstores. For further information, call 800-337-2665 or visit our website at www.northatlanticbooks.com.

Substantial discounts on bulk quantities are available to corporations, professional associations, and other organizations. For details and discount information, contact our special sales department.

Library of Congress Cataloging-in-Publication Data

Schwab, Sidney M., 1944-
    Cutting remarks : insights and recollections of a surgeon / by Sidney M. Schwab.
        p. ; cm.
    Includes index.
    Summary: "A prominent surgeon's reflections on his medical training and profession, a nuanced, behind-the scenes picture of modern medicine and how doctors relate to both their peers and their patients. Above all a portrait of the kind of character it takes to be a surgeon"—Provided by the publisher.
    ISBN 1-58394-147-9 (trade paper)
    1. Schwab, Sidney M., 1944- 2. Surgeons—United States—Biography.
    [DNLM: 1. Schwab, Sidney M., 1944- 2. Surgery—Personal Narratives. WZ 100 S398s 2006] I. Title.
    RD27.35.S385A3 2006
    617.092—dc22

                                                          2005033140
                                                              CIP

        1 2 3 4 5 6 7 8 9 UNITED 10 09 08 07 06

Dedication

For Mom and Dad
Don't worry. It was a long time ago.

For Judy
Thanks for putting up with it; then, and now.

For Dan
You make me proud.

and

For my mentors
May they rest in peace.
Especially the ones that aren't dead yet.

Contents

Part Three: The Beginning

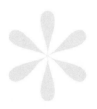

Reality Check

Someone said writing is easy: you just sit down at a typewriter and open a vein. As I've been in the business of preventing bleeding, this may not work out well. You wouldn't want John Updike taking out your gallbladder.

Introduction

A surgeon can kill you. Other doctors, to whom it doesn't come as naturally, need a sustained and concerted effort, and even then they might have a hard time. But surgeons do it as quickly and easily as the flash of an operating light on sharpened steel, and you'll sleep right through it. Surgical residency is the process by which a freshly hatched, still-quivering medical student is turned into someone for whom you'd lie on a table and spread open your belly—an optimistic venture for teacher, student, and of course you.

This is a memoir, along with the occasional reflection and explanation, of my general surgery internship and residency, from 1970 to 1977, at The University of California, San Francisco. In that era, surgical training required encompassing commitment: round-the-clock work hours were expected for days on end. Until only a few years earlier, UCSF had refused to accept anyone who was married.

The Chairman of Surgery at UCSF in the early seventies was J. Englebert ("Bert") Dunphy, one of a tight group of surgeons that had trained together at Harvard and spent World War II operating in tents around Europe, having, by their accounts, a great time. They came home and spread across America, eventually heading some of the country's best surgery programs. Giants—the school in "old school." (The "old" too, by the time I got there.)

Dr. Dunphy expected total immersion in training, believed in the learning value of working day and night, cut through all the excuses people made for their screw-ups, and was a great teacher. He also had an omnipresent sense of humor and an explosive laugh, most commonly heard after telling his own jokes. (Example: He told us that as an intern, making rounds in Boston, he presented a burn victim: "This man set himself on fire from smoking in bed." "I resent that!" the man shouted. "That bed was on fire when I got into it!") His hand was firm, but he had a way of making us happy to eat out of it. Being around him was a rare treat; he spent lots of time away, as guest professor all over the world.

I told myself a million times that I should be writing things down and of course never did. So here I am conjuring up a time long past. Some memories come easily. Others draw blood. In the process of recollection, I realize how much great stuff has been lost forever, and I have decided not to fill in those blank spots with fiction. I won't testify to the certainty of chronology; nor, if you were to pry open my head and pick through the lost data, can I say you'd find that each story happened exactly as I told it. Age does that. On the other hand, those people and events that stuck with me must have done so for a reason.

Patient names are made up. So are those of many doctors, mainly the ones I might have cast in unflattering light. Those whose imprints are positive and long-lasting are truly named: Dunphy, Blaisdell, Richards, Utley, Goldstone, Trunkey, Schrock. Several others. They are part of who I am, surgically speaking. Nor were the others entirely negative: no encounter during my training passed without meaning. Learning what not to do is no less important than figuring out what's right.

I recall and have recorded failures more than successes, probably because good outcomes were expected and rarely acknowledged, and because disaster is the better teacher. That you made a mistake was announced in private, on rounds, and in front of the combined gathering of every surgeon at UCSF. It could be blistering. I've always had that view, anyway; it took me many years in practice even to acknowledge thank-yous, much less think they were deserved. Like most surgeons, I beat myself up when anything was less than perfect with my patients. Surgical training in those days was the ideal way to have such an outlook reinforced. With a blowtorch.

Some historical perspective: "Intern" is an antiquated medical term. Since practically no one practices medicine anymore without at least two years of specialty training, the first year is now called R-1 (for "resident, level one"), and R-2, R-3, and so on identify the subsequent years of training. But in the '70s we began as interns, heirs to tradition. And there was a time when the chief resident position was more of an honor than it was by the time I got there. You didn't have to serve as chief resident to go out and ply your wares; the chiefship was optional, neither given out nor taken lightly. It lay somewhere between trainee and professor. In my time, it had become more of a fancy name for the last year of training than a special honor. Nevertheless, not every surgical resident who sought to become a fully trained surgeon at UCSF was able to do so. The axe, if it were to fall, did so after the second or third year of residency, sometimes brutally. Lots of bodies were needed to do the grunt work of patient care in the various hospitals; but by the time it comes to topping off brains and rendering them fully trained, you can't spread the experience among a dozen people. Some headed elsewhere naturally, to various surgical subspecialties that require only a couple of years of general surgery

Cutting Remarks

training. Others got shunted into the lab for an extra year. Some just got summarily left behind and had to find another program in which to finish. Making it to the top, on occasion, meant a certain amount of resident blood had been spilled.

Internship and residency have always been a curious mix of structure on the outside and chaos within. At a given institution, the makeup of each year is specified in terms of way-stations on the road to knowledge: interns and residents rotate serially through various services and specialties. But within those services there's no spelled-out list of requirements, no boxes to check. Time is defined, but not texture. You show up at a certain hospital location on a given day, spend your month, or two, or four. And after the last day, you show up somewhere else and start again. What you get out of it depends on a serendipitous coming together of your own mettle, the mix of patients that happen to pass through, and the teaching proclivities and talents of the professors. No one officially measures what you learned until it's all over. (I took exams to become certifed by the American Board of Surgery, and had to provide lists of operations done and undergo interviews and get supporting references to become a Fellow of the American College of Surgeons. But there were no exams at any point in the training at UCSF.) Some interns and residents might, on a particular service, do several hernia repairs, others none. Some well, some badly. Evaluation, to the extent that it occurred, was covert and mysteri-

UCSF is a very academically oriented program. Many surgical residents had professorships in mind, and did a year of research in the process of training. Some took that third year and went abroad—mainly England—to do a clinical year. Getting back out into the mainstream sometimes was tough, if you were considered a marginal candidate for the gold ring, or if—as sometimes occurred—there were more hot candidates than they could find room for in a given year.

ous. I recall being asked my opinion about junior residents when I was a senior. I don't know what role, if any, those opinions played, nor did I get general feedback on my own performance. For a given situation, teaching points might be made, criticism or praise handed out; but there was never a formalized review of my progress that I saw, no end-of-the-year report. Each year, I was allowed to continue, with no explanations given. "Metrics," in the Rumsfeldian sense, did not exist then; they are, however, being addressed in a more rational way currently. Labs, for example, have been devised to test certain surgical skills without the need for human subjects.

Another thing: "general surgeon." The term doesn't seem to have the cachet of "brain surgeon." Fact is, a general surgeon is what every surgeon used to be: one who did it all. Now, various specialties have taken their bag of tricks and slunk away: neurosurgery, orthopedics, urology, gynecology. More than leftovers, general surgery remains the most diverse of the surgical specialties and requires the broadest knowledge: we care for thyroids, parathyroids, breasts, livers, gallbladders, pancreases, esophagi, stomachs, spleens, small and large intestines, appendices, adrenals, hernias, hemorrhoids, and more. Most cancer surgery is done by general surgeons. And, unlike the majority of other surgical sub-specialties, we like to manage the entire person in whom those organs are packaged. *"A general surgeon is an internist who can operate."* That's the mantra we heard in training. An orthopedist calls for help when a patient needs fluid management, and will run screaming out of the room if there's a need for diabetic

"Internist" is shorthand for a specialist in internal medicine. An "intern" is a doctor in the first year of training after medical school. In the latter case, I'd guess the name derives from a similar word used to describe being held prisoner.

control. A general surgeon hitches up the pants (or panties) and goes to work.

✳

There may have been a certain trial-by-fire hazing aspect to training in my day, but it was also believed—by trainer and trainee alike—that this was the only way to produce a person with the knowledge, skill, and commitment to keep patients safe. They might have been right. If so, a trail of corpses will lead us to the truth in a few years; the 120- to 140-hour work week we faced back then has (since around 2000, resulting from a lawsuit in New York City) been cut to a pathetic, embarrassing, and paltry 80 hours now.

OK, so things have changed some since training days. Now we have intensivists and hospitalists: medical docs who do nothing but care for critically ill or even routinely hospitalized patients, including post-ops. For surgeons, that's partly from needing to do more and more operations, as reimbursement has declined by over half, with less and less time to manage all care; second, it has to do with liability issues; and, third, it's not an entirely bad thing to have super-sick people cared for by docs who do nothing but that sort of thing. Ignoring the vision of Dr. Dunphy shifting uncomfortably in his grave, I'll say that critically ill patients get better care now from an intensivist. Most general surgeons still feel like handling routine medical needs, and staying involved in the ICU. Ortho, neuro? "Call me when they go home or die."

thanks

Acknowledgments

In the introduction I said that some memories drew blood. The main lubricant of the process was, in fact, honey. I have several people to thank. English professor and college roomie Al Powers gave wise and witty advice. English teacher and sister-in-law Janet Mumma gave valuable time early in the process. Attorney, teacher, author, and friend Jennie Heard freely gave not only encouragement but also incisive proofreading. Kathy Glass did, too, though not so freely. And I'm quite amazed that Richard Grossinger of North Atlantic Books/Frog, Ltd., took a chance on a novice writer; his generous and thorough notes had much to do with the shape of the final version. Julie Brand, also of NAB/Frog, has been virtuously patient with my nearly constant flow of emails.

Medical men gave much: both Jerry Goldstone and Bill Schecter—each of them more than busy enough as academic surgeons and leaders—provided brain-jogging recollections. In a contest among surgical professors for nicest, hardest-working, most modest in the face of great accomplishment and respect from peers, they'd finish in a dead heat, at the head of the pack. (Not much of a contest, really, using "nice" and "modest" as criteria for judging surgeons.)

I make special mention of Dr. F. William Blaisdell (thirty years later, I still can't call him "Bill") and feel the need specifically to

Cutting Remarks

acknowledge his reservations. He said he mostly liked the book a lot but he had real concerns that I had cast UCSF in a bad light and was not convinced by my arguments to the contrary. My respect for the Blazer is boundless, as it is for UCSF; I only hope he will see that whereas my gratitude and love for the training I had is not entirely blind, it is profound. Had I the chance to do it all over again, God help me, I would.

Finally, of course, there is Judy. She dog-paddled back into my life in the California gold country and stayed firmly put, only to have to listen to me reading aloud line after line, over and over, thirty-five years later. What a girl!

part

The Start

one

one

Inklings

Looking around at a sea of suits, crested here and there with curls of white coats bobbing in slumber, I have an idea. It's Saturday morning at the end of a long week, and I've been at the podium for a few minutes, feeling the usual mix of confidence and nakedness, in front of a collection of professors, residents, and students. As chief resident on the Gold Service at UCSF hospital, I am presenting data at our weekly "D and C" (for Death and Complication) Conference. In a large and overly-warm auditorium, I've made it through a humdrum list of complications with only a couple of questions thrown at me. Easy. There's a bit of a problem case to explain, but I think I might be able to sneak it by. "The death occurred in a seventy-two-year-old woman, with multiple admissions for chronic pancreatitis, enterocutaneous fistula, and Korsakoff's psychosis," I say. (The lady had an inflamed pancreas, intestinal juices draining out through her skin, and alcohol-related dementia.) "On this admission," I go on, "she was found to have a new fistula, pancreatic insufficiency, and bilateral pneumonia. At the request of her family, she was given comfort measures only, had a gradual downhill course, caught fire, and died." Waiting a beat, I look down at the lectern while still trying to peek at the audience. Nothing. I make ready to continue, but Jack Wylie, the professor leading the conference, leans my way, scowls up one eyebrow, and says, "Caught fire?" Damn. I'm going to have to explain. And I will. Later.

Seven years earlier, I'd begun my surgical training on the Blue Service (blue and gold, University of California colors), one of about a dozen rotations at four hospitals through which I'd be passing several times, as intern, junior (two years' worth) and senior resident, finally chief resident. UC Moffitt, San Francisco General Hospital, the VA, Children's. Trauma, elective, extremity, private, pediatrics, transplant, cardiac, the burn unit, and more. I showed up about a week after getting my medical degree, another of many trips I'd taken up and down the totem pole over the past twenty-six years. This was the most slippery slide from eagle to turtle. "Congratulations, doctor," I heard with pride as I was handed my MD degree in Cleveland. "Shave your beard and get your ass to 6A tomorrow at five a.m." was the suggestion in San Francisco. I was there at 4:45, expecting some sort of orientation. There's the call room, here's where we keep the charts, the lab's downstairs. ... What happened was that Walt R., the outgoing intern—who looked like he'd fallen off his camel a week ago and dragged himself through the desert—handed me some cards with patient names, said "Good luck with the Judge," and staggered off, as if toward a shimmering cooler of beer. Wendell P. showed up, the other intern on the service. A few minutes later, so did the chief resident, a couple of junior residents, and a med student or two. I willed myself through the wall of heat and stepped into a cauldron, the approach to which had begun several years earlier.

✳

My dad and aunt were lawyers; I labeled myself "pre-law" on

my college applications but was also mindful that my biological father, who died before I was born, was a doctor. Inspired by reading letters his patients sent when he died, I took some pre-med courses at Amherst and soon realized that I was having more fun in labs than in libraries. For example, when my lab partner set our chemistry experiment on fire and reacted by opening a drawer full of lab books and sweeping in the burning goo, we were able to laugh (after determining that the books were salvageable). Had that happened in the Robert Frost Library, we'd probably still be in jail.

My senior honors thesis was on the ruby-eye mutation of *Drosophila melanogaster* (fruit fly). Since those bugs start fornicating within hours of birth, I frequently had to wake up in the wee hours and head to the lab to separate them before they contaminated the gene pool; at the time, I thought of it as parenting. I see now that it was preparation for being on call. Unable to make a soulful connection to flies, I nevertheless dedicated the thesis to Ray Charles, quoting his line, "They say, Ruby, you're like a dream, not always what you seem," which—seer that he was—predicted the results I presented.

Before my senior year at Amherst, sitting in the office of Cactus Jack Caughey, the admissions dean at Western Reserve University in Cleveland (now Case-Western Reserve), I heard

Cactus Jack's name was aptly nicked. Bullet-shaped and gruffly voiced, he was a one-man admissions committee, in fact if not on paper. Students loved him despite his apparent severity. This was during the Vietnam War, and our class was not shy about political activism. Hell, we even sent our freebie doctor bags back to Eli Lilly, the first group in the country to do so. At a meeting in which we were discussing a moratorium on classes to protest the war, Jack stormed in and said, "What we need is a moratorium on bullshit." He also liked to ask prospective students why they wanted to be a doctor. When he heard the predictable answer— "because I like people"—he'd ask, "Yes, but do you like sick people?"

him rumble, "We'll take ya," after which I flew my shiny new '65 Mustang a few feet off the ground and headed back to college for my final year which, unburdened as it was from medical school admissions worry, was a fine one, indeed. When I returned to Cleveland, I was excited and hopeful, tempered only by the race riots that had broken out in the city and the fact that Jim Brown had announced his retirement from football. On the other hand, while I was there the Cuyahoga River burned—an event immortalized in song by Randy Newman. The constant target of jokes ("First prize: a week in Cleveland. Second prize: two weeks"), Cleveland was not entirely bad.

What made Western Reserve a highly sought-after school, in those days, was the fact that it had dramatically changed the age-old, time-weary approach of studying by category; anatomy, physiology, biochemistry. At Reserve, subjects were grouped by organ system; so we studied the anatomy, physiology, etc, of the cardiovascular system, or the digestive system. Logical, yet revolutionary. We also had some exposure to patients right away, which reminded us why we were actually there. We were each assigned a family, in which the wife was pregnant. We took calls in the night, made house calls, attended the birth. They called us "doctor." Call in the middle of the night: (Patient:) the baby won't sleep. (Me:) I'll get back to you. (Me:) the baby won't sleep. (Attending:) does he have a fever? (Me:) I'll get back to you. . . .

As is well-known from other medical school tales, the first two years of the four are mostly devoted to book-learning: lectures and labs, not much patient contact. It wasn't until we got to the third year that we were full-time in the hospitals, seeing actual people. The TV show "ER" to the contrary, med students don't know much, and do less. I found it unrewarding to be the fifth or sixth person to poke his finger up a patient's rear end, knowing that he knew that I had no clue what I was doing. Even when I did, it was irrelevant to the actual care of that patient; he was doing me a service, not the other way around.

So I was thrilled when I found myself on the surgery rotation at Cleveland Metropolitan General Hospital. It was my good luck that John Davis, who was the Chief of Surgery—highly respected there and around the country—had announced his planned departure the following year. As a result, the surgery training program had signed up no interns, so med students were designated "acting interns" (irony aside) and found themselves a necessary part of the team. What we did was useful, of all things, and we got the occasional bone of gratitude thrown to us: we sometimes got to do little surgical procedures. "Do" is a deceptive term. Deftly moving a patient around under him, it's possible to have a student hold a knife and think he did something, the operation proceeding without the student knowing what the hell just happened. Usually, this meant removing a cyst or something pretty simple. But I was allowed to "do" a hernia repair. Scared and thrilled, my hand shook enough that it was probably visible across the hall, but I cut through the skin in one stroke (nothing worse than seeing a neophyte scratch and scratch at the skin, leaving parallel marks that barely bleed), didn't do anything stupid, and got to the end feeling epiphanized. Not that I understood the mechanics of what I'd just done; but I knew that something had resonated. The feeling grabbed me, a palpable validation, a come-on.

On my last day of the rotation, I was taking the afternoon off when I got a page from the senior resident, announcing one more great case for me to do—would I come back in? Mustang flying past Lake Erie once again, I headed back to CMGH. The patient was a derelict diabetic, found under a bridge, with one leg half dead, needing radical debridement (cutting away dead tissue). He was already in the OR, prepped and draped, by the time I got there. Swollen, blistered, and stinking, only the leg was visible, with maggots grazing between the toes. The resident handed me the knife and showed me where to cut. Which I did, liberating the most foul stuff I'd ever seen or smelled. Nauseating sewage, it ran down the leg onto my shoes and the floor. I wondered if calling me in had been a final gift to a respected student, or a reminder that I was just a grunt, after all. Or that surgeons could be jerks. I'm still not sure, the last two possibilities definitely being true.

Disgusting as that sounds, I came to realize a surgical fact: if draining something stinks up the whole OR and makes the people in it want to vomit, it's definitely a good thing for the patient. Not universally true of all operations.

There had been another discovery in med school: dog labs. I'd always had dogs—I love dogs—including Buttons, the world's smartest. Doing experiments on them was something about which I had very mixed feelings. There would be an animal for every four of us, each dog lying on our regular lab tables, already asleep. There were smells, and there was guilt, and at the end, the dogs would be dumped into plastic bags and carted off. But I found it fascinating, inside a belly, handling warm living tissues. Clamping, tying, cutting. Badly, but still. . . .

The following summer, I got a fellowship to work in a lab back home in Oregon, with Albert Starr, inventor of the first widely successful artificial heart valve. I saw Dr. Starr only once: he came into the lab one Monday and asked his research assistant what he'd done over the weekend. "Worked in the yard," he said. "You did WHAT??" Al shrieked. He held up his hands, fingers spread. "See these? Each one of these fingers is worth a million dollars to me. [note: 1967 dollars] You think I'd risk them working in the yard?" I thought to myself, yeah, but. . . . I worked with several of Dr.

Starr's research fellows, who were testing valves and a lung-substitute device by implanting them in dogs. In the process, I got handy with a couple of surgical techniques, including gaining access to the carotid artery (in the neck, supplying blood to the brain) through a very small incision. Not long after returning to school, there was another dog lab; this one required placing pressure monitors directly into the carotid (coincidence, or karma?). Such experiments depend, among other things, on not causing too much trauma prior to collecting data. Since the other students were coming up with lots of useless data, when the prof noticed how easily I'd gotten to the carotid on my dog, I ended up exposing carotids for each group, admiration following me as I moved modestly from table to table. Such are the rewards of being able to do something, a surgical virtue if ever there was one.

Of my medical school memories, next to those surgical the strongest are the ones from my psychiatry rotation, especially memories of talking to schizophrenics. All were young adults who seemed to have a depth and breadth of intelligence that far outstripped my own and that led me to believe that their craziness came from seeing, more than anyone else, the world as it really is; and that the clarity was too much for them. If, I thought, we could puzzle our way into their brains, we could find TRUTH, though surely we'd not want to. I got more positive feedback on the psych rotation than from any other, including surgery: they wondered if I really wanted to be a surgeon. It was a waste, they thought, because I was so good at talking to people. But I think talking surgeons have helped at least as many people as talking shrinks.

When it came time to apply for internships, I had no hesitation in choosing surgery. Despite its reputation for being more demanding than any other program, UCSF was my first choice. It was considered to be among the top two or three in the country (guess you'll have to take my word for it). Knowing I'd have a job in Cleveland, I interviewed at several places across the country feeling unpressured, and I had what felt like good encounters with several UCSF profs. Western Reserve didn't have class rankings (another of its innovations—wonder if it's still true). With undisguised anger, the chief of another program had asked, "Why should I choose you, with no class rank, over someone from, oh, Michigan who's tenth in his class?" "Because there's more to judging a doctor than a number?" (I didn't really want to go there, anyway.) No one at UCSF brought it up. I hoped my recommendations and interviews would be enough.

Internship acceptance letters came out all at once (there was a complicated computerized nationwide matching program) and were sent to the medical schools. Talk about a bizarre scene: at Reserve, the entire class sat in a lecture hall while names were called and the internships announced out loud. People went up to the podium to receive their paperwork, some elated, some crestfallen, some struggling to look impassive, to the occasional murmur of the others. Everyone knew what the hot jobs were. I was pleased when my name was called.

Toward the end of internship I was asked to sit on an application review committee. It was revelatory. It's amazing how many applications looked the same, all fabulous. Letters of recommendation were key. You could easily tell the boilerplate items: "This is an excellent student who will do well wherever he goes." The ones that stood out were those that said "this is the finest student I've seen in twenty years," and gave examples. The salutation was important, too. "Dear Dr. Dunphy" was adequate. "Dear Dr. Englebert" of which there were a couple, missed the mark. "Dear Bert" went into a separate pile. I know I got a "Dear Bert" letter out of my time in Oregon, where Dr. Dunphy had been chief before he went to SF.

two

Into the Blue

Fellow intern Wendell and I were trailing the entourage heading toward the ICU (intensive care unit) to meet the first, and sickest, of our patients. This one day of the year, patient information was presented to the new interns. After that, we were expected to know and to pass the information to the more senior residents, who would grill us, sometimes teach us, and assign work for the day. In those days of the iron men (and the rare woman) we were expected to draw the blood for tests, start the IVs, collect lab data, produce X-rays for viewing, place tubes into various orifices, admit and discharge the patients, handle the paperwork, write orders, scrub into the operations, respond to calls from the nurses. The UCSF surgical program was tough: the lighter rotations were those in which there were two interns, which meant we got every other night off (after a 36- to 40-hour stretch), and every other weekend. On the harder ones there was only one intern. That could mean twelve out of fourteen days straight in the hospital, and the weekend on call required covering an additional and unfamiliar service from which another lone intern had gotten sprung for the weekend. Time off started mid-afternoon on Saturday, after patient rounds and D and C conference, and ended around five a.m. Monday morning.

So we're standing in the ICU, hearing about the Judge. An actual judge, as it turns out, from Northern California, in the hospital for weeks. Belly bloated, skin thin and pasty, tube from nose draining gallons of intestinal juices each day, he'd undergone countless operations, the original for forgotten reasons, and subsequent ones for innumerable bowel obstructions. The surgical implications were way over my head; my problem was going to be keeping track of the unheard-of amounts of fluids leaking out of him, along with the electrolytes (salts) they contained, and trying to replace them without killing him in the process. The Judge's private doc was Phillip Griswold. The slick, the silver-haired, the sweet-smelling. His locker in the OR had a full shelf of powders, oils, and unguents of various types, with which, while gazing admiringly into a mirror, he regularly abluted himself, slowly, taking in the view, liking what he was seeing. Smooth and elegant, he always sat on a patient's bed, held the wrist in a grand gesture and appeared to feel the pulse as he spoke. Mellifluous. Fatherly. A mediocre surgeon, but an accomplished operator. It seemed—later, as I began to understand such things—that the last few operations on the Judge might have been ill-advised. What was apparent was that his bowel was lying within him and not moving, digestive juices backing up; the explanation was (and remains) unclear. There was reason to believe he had some unspecified and undiagnosable dysfunction of his gut, such that by now he might never regain enough intestinal activity to handle his own juices. No one had ever seen so much drainage, of such unusual chemical makeup. Not me, sure as hell.

In the next bed was Carol Bates. Seventyish, prim, sweet-smiling. She'd had aggressive radiation therapy to her neck and the center of her chest and had been cooked from the inside out. Her aorta, the main artery from her heart, was peeling away its outer layers like a bad sunburn. (Radiation technique has come a long way since those days.) She'd been to the OR several times in the last weeks, her surgeons tying off yet another squirting arterial branch, and was now at the point where the next leak would be her last. Unable to talk but fully alert, she spent much of her time looking in a compact mirror as she dabbed with a tissue or cleansed with a Q-tip, tending to the hole in her neck that was the end of her trachea—the upper part having long since rotted away. Mrs. Bates handled her own suction device. It was my distinct impression that she didn't know she'd run out of options.

Outside the ICU, things were not so grim. There was a reassuring assortment of post-op patients, recovering well from routine procedures on their gallbladders, colons, breasts, groins, ani. Nothing scary. But now it was time to head to the OR, to scrub with surgeons I'd not yet met, on patients I did not yet know, but who'd be—at some level—my responsibility later in the day. Thus began the endless loop of lots to do, with little time to do it.

Every pretend doc you ever see, on every TV show you ever watch, contaminates him- or herself a dozen times in full view of the cameras, between washing and getting gowned and gloved, not to mention when they play around with instruments. (Note to Hollywood: I'm available.) Fresh interns are fair game in the operating room, for everyone, starting with the scrub nurses. Amused and even sympathetic toward students, nurses were ruthless with interns: the slightest breach, real or not, and back you'd go to the sink to start over. It was a major accomplishment to wash, rinse, towel off, don the gown and gloves without touching something, dropping hands too low, forgetting the mask before starting. And then getting the drapes properly placed on the patient, appropriate for the operation to be done and the peculiar preferences of the surgeon doing it, not touching them to something unsterile, just so. (Now there are disposable paper drapes, shaped just right for any given operation. Back then, we used sterile cloth sheets, of which there were several required for each operation: various shapes and sizes, laid here and there to cover and expose, and each surgeon had a different idea of the exactly correct way to do it.) It seemed impossible ever to figure it all out, and this was only soap, water, and a bunch of cloth. The scratch on the scratch of the surface. To know how long is the journey, and to find yourself unable even to locate your shoes—those first few days in the OR were demoralizing to the point of intestinal dysfunction.

You'd think the operating room would be the center of a surgery intern's world. In fact, since we did little and often couldn't see much, it could be a major pain—several hours during which work was piling up, and because of which sleep that night was receding further into impossibility. Shifting weight from one foot to the other, ignoring the aches in the back of the knees, holding hooks, often in both hands, straining beyond trembling of the arms and shoulders, we were grilled about the disease, the procedure, the anatomy in question. What's this vessel? Tell me the circulation to the transverse colon. What's behind this that I could injure? Or, just as likely: hold this retractor. Pull. Can you see ok? Yes, sir. Then you're not pulling hard enough.

Yet always there was the hope that someone would hand me a knife and

My father-in-law has a great story in this regard from his training: a fellow intern, having been sent back to re-scrub many times, finally made it to the table just as the surgeon was calling for a particular clamp. "Kelley," the surgeon ordered, hand out. The intern took the hand and shook it. "Albertson," he responded, proudly. (Proving the surgeons-can-be-jerks truism, the surgeon tossed the intern out of the OR.)

let me make an incision. Let me learn the tension needed to expose an area, allow me to place a clamp, tie a knot. Cutting suture was the interns' uncontested domain. With a flourish of generosity, the surgeon would ask us to cut the suture he'd just tied. Pathetic. So trivial; yet we strove for perfection. Touch the knot with the blade of the scissor, turn it just so, and cut. Usually followed by "too short!" or "too long!" The harsh glare of the nurses, the other surgeons, making one want to ask the next time, "Do you want this one too short or too long, doctor?" But maybe I'd get the chance to put my hand around and behind the liver, learning how it feels, how to expose it. Sneak into that hidden space behind the right colon, or the one behind the stomach. Cut between a pair of clamps. Ten seconds out of thirty-six hours' straight work was all it took. It happened about once a week. Enough to keep us going, to remind us why we were there. Enough to motivate us to steal suture from the OR and practice tying knots. Chairs in the work areas were hairy with suture around the rungs, dangling slip knots, surgeons' knots, tied one-handed, two-handed, overhand, underhand. I carried around a surgical clamp, having gotten into the habit of locking and unlocking it, over and over, using my palm, not my fingers. The cool way. For all the years I was there, the clamp hung inside my white coat, to be fiddled with on rounds, unconsciously.

Heading back to the surgical floor after a few hours in the OR, I would—for weeks—confront doubt and fear: so much to know, so much to do, so many years to go. In fact, especially with surgery, the training of a doctor is anything but a lonely process. It's top-down; the chain of command gets established clearly and repeated often. An intern may be the first responder, but he's hardly alone. UCSF surgery in the seventies was, as far as we could tell, the program in the US where interns were allowed the least freedom and did the fewest operations. Every decision was checked with the next-level resident, who likely checked with the next higher. No non-private patient went to the OR without having discussed the case with an attending professor; except for pretty mundane operations, the attending was likely to be present in the room. And so it was for patient care on the floors. The intern was usually first to see the patient, but a junior resident was always close and, mostly, sympathetic. Not so much a matter of feeling like I'd do something wrong, my angst was more about wondering if I'd ever get to the point of being able to do this stuff on my own.

Going to my first D and C conference didn't help: here were the chief residents of every service in every hospital reporting their week. To watch the trauma chief from SFGH was to see into a world so daunting and distant as to seem forever out of reach. After the chiefs of the other services described twenty or twenty-five admissions, fifteen or twenty operations, no deaths, a couple of complications, the trauma chief strode to the podium and announced seventy admissions, eighty operations (Wondering about the math? Trauma patients very often require more than one operation.), seven deaths, nineteen complications. And he went through each death, each complication: an eight-story jumper, a kid run over by a MUNI bus, a victim of a point-blank .357 Magnum. Chest opened and aorta clamped in the ER, taken to the OR, liver partly resected, six holes in the bowel repaired, kidney removed. Got a wound infection. Imagining myself in that position, calmly and confidently having handled such things, was beyond possible. But what an irresistible goal! Could it ever be me doing that? I told myself several times a day, "Everyone went through it, everyone started just the same."

*

I got more of the lowdown on the Judge. The immediate problem would be maintaining fluid and electrolyte balance. Samples of his drainage were sent daily to the lab to measure the electrolyte composition, and solutions were prepared with additives to give it all back. To replace lost acid, the mixture he was getting had so much ammonium chloride in it that it smelled like cleaning fluid. Having passed not even the suggestion of a fart or feces in weeks, the man nevertheless showed no intestinal blockage on his X-rays. Another operation, in other words, would be of no use. Over the next several days I got comfortable figuring out what he needed in his IV (IV stands for IntraVenous, a needle or tube in a vein—or the medications or fluids going through it), but there was no end in sight; no one really knew what was going on. The Judge got to me; my dad was a judge. The two seemed to share an unjudicial temperament of impatience. Although the Judge was not always fully alert, I could sense his deep desire to get fixed or get gone. No metaphor: shit or get off the planet. There was a new class of drugs—commonplace now, not much used then—which directly reduced the acid output of the stomach. It occurred to me that using such a drug in his IV might cut back on the acid and maybe even the amount of fluid he needed. (A lightning bolt then, this idea has become routine now.) Dr. Griswold had long since run out of ideas, so he was perfectly ok with it. Couldn't have cared less, actually. Probably hoping we'd bump him off, so he could blame someone.

Miraculous. A significant drop in output, and a return to more normal acid balance. Over the next few days, with the output from his stomach tube diminishing, I wondered what would happen if we stopped suction on the tube—maybe we were chasing our tail: suck it out, drip it back in. The amount coming out after turning the suction back on wasn't higher, which suggested that fluid was moving downstream. We started using the suction more and more intermittently and finally I just yanked the tube. Not only did he not get more bloated, the Judge started pooping by the bedfull. He'd been getting some nutrients in his IVs, but now we could risk trying food. There's a stimulative effect of food in the gut. A paradox in this case: can't feed him while he's bloated; can't get rid of the bloat without feeding him. So we began gingerly to fuel the Judge with the real thing, and for the first time in a couple of months, there was a light flickering. Now I was determined to get him home. He'd been bedridden for weeks; physical therapists weren't available then as they are now, so it was up to me

"Better to be lucky than good"—another surgical dictum.

to get him out of bed. It took convincing: he was listless and weak. But I struggled him upright on the side of his bed, draped him over my shoulders, and stood him up. He was, it turned out, a giant. I'm six-feet-four (was, back then) and he towered over me.

We had another mystery patient: she'd undergone routine intestinal surgery, was making a normal recovery, but every time we'd start her on food, she'd vomit. Back would go the stomach tube, things would proceed to the point of apparent readiness to eat, tube out, feed, vomit, tube in. . . . Finally we asked Dr. Dunphy what he thought was going on. "What are you feeding her?" he asked. Clear liquids. The routine first meal after surgery. Jello, broth. "Give her a steak!" he said. Gotta be kidding, right? "How would you like to be looking at green jello when you feel crummy? Give her a steak." We did. She gobbled it up, and went home. When I went into my own practice, I almost never ordered clear liquids post-op.

If he collapsed, it would have been monumental; but we managed a couple of steps.

"C'mon, Judge. Left foot, right foot, left foot, right foot. . . ."

"Left, right, left, right," he coughed.

"You're doing great, Judge. Left, right, way to go, left, right, way to go. . . ."

"Left, right, go to hell, left, right, go to hell," he said.

A couple of weeks later, we watched medics wheel the Judge to a waiting air-ambulance, and he made it back to Redwood City. For about a week. He came back—bloated, in respiratory failure—and died a few days later. Dr. Griswold made me be the one to take him off the ventilator. His private patient, whom I'd come to like and admire, and whose brief escape to home was my proud accomplishment. "Pull the plug," Griswold said, and walked off. Bastard.

Pretty soon it was two for two. Carol Bates, the other original ICU patient, had been moved to a private room on the floor. No point in taking up critical space. Playing a kind of musical night call, each morning I'd ask Wendell, or he'd ask me, if Carol had made it through the night; and she'd be there, calmly dabbing her open throat, suctioning her trachea hole, reading. Rouge on her cheeks, hair neatly combed. Waiting. "Hello, Mrs. Bates, how are you today?" She'd smile. "Anything you need?" She'd shake her head. "You're looking good, you're doing good." Check her bandages, look at her neck, and off to the next room. She lasted another couple of weeks. And then, at night, with me the one on duty, her call light went on while I was at the nurses' station. I ran into her room as she turned to me with fear in her fading eyes, rouged sweat running down her cheeks, making all the more obvious her evolving pallor. "It's ok, it's ok," I said, sitting on her bed, taking her wrist, as if feeling her pulse.

three

Blood on the Walls

Lester Weisman looked like Death. Bony, stooped, hook-nosed, and spider-fingered, he spoke in a voice that was chronically hoarse, a wheezing gust from Hades. He walked slowly, head down, peering above his glasses. Raising a hand toward you if he addressed you, he let the fingers droop and motioned vaguely, as if it were too much effort to point. When he smiled, it looked like he smelled something putrid. He should have carried a scythe, but it would have been unseemly for a former chairman of the department.

I liked him a lot. At this point in his career he had only a few patients, but he gave the occasional lecture. "The parathyroid . . . [grimace] . . . was first described . . . [sigh] . . . in the African water buffaloooh . . . [lengthy exhale]. . . ." Weisman even still did the occasional thyroid or parathyroid operation, and I wondered what his patients thought when they met him: hoarseness is the main complication of such operations, and he was the anthropomorphism of the word. In the OR, I watched him say, "I can't see a goddamn thing. It's too dark . . . Aim the light here, goddammit . . . No, HERE! . . . Goddamn it . . . OK, turn off the goddamn lights, all of them. Turn 'em OFF. . . Now turn on that one. THAT ONE! . . . [cough] . . . Now aim it RIGHT HERE godDAMN it!!" Amusing.

One of Dr. Weisman's relatives, a powerful local executive, was admitted in a hurry, vomiting blood. Lester shepherded the care, standing nervously and helplessly aside while a gastroenterologist tried to get a scope into the stomach, looking for the source (difficult when there's lots of blood). Finally, after witnessing his relative retching non-stop, struggling against the sedatives, and continuing to bleed, Lester said, "That's enough, we're going to the OR." As the intern on the case, with all the more senior people otherwise engaged, I was the main assistant. Such bleeding—GI bleeding (for gastrointestinal), as we call it—is much less common nowadays, given the better treatments for ulcers; and when there is a GI bleed, often you can avoid emergency surgery with various other interventions. In the majority of cases, when surgery is needed, it's known pretty accurately where the problem is. In this case, with no history of prior bleeding or causative factors, and a failed endoscopy, it was going to be a crap-shoot. Nor was the patient in optimum shape; ideally you'd like to get the tank refilled with blood and fluid, because when anesthesia begins, the body's natural responses to low volume are suppressed. Blood pressure that's been maintained by various stress responses can drop like a frightened intern's face. Which it did. Having already broken a cardinal rule and taken on the care of a close relative, Lester had also rushed him to the OR before adequate resuscitation. When the bleeding is brisk enough, there may be no choice. Had it not been his kin, I think Dr. Weisman would have taken the extra time. The anesthesiologist had his hands full for a while, and I squeezed in a couple of pints of blood before scrubbing into the case. The crash was not fatal, but it added to the sense of pressure and dread. And portended a tough recovery.

Not knowing the exact source of bleeding, one plays the odds and makes the first gastric incision at the lower end, across the pylorus (control muscle at the bottom of the stomach), where statistics say most bleeding occurs. Sometimes it's right there: a spurting artery on the back side of the stomach or duodenum (the first part of the small intestine, starting at the bottom end of the stomach), pumping impressively but accessible without difficulty. A couple of big sutures and it's over. Not today. We saw fresh blood, clots, bits of food, but no obvious source of the bleeding. Dr. Weisman's silence filled the room like a cold fog as he made another cut, higher up the stomach, closer to the esophagus. It's hard getting all the way up there; the esophagus comes into the belly at the back, and you're operating from the front, with the ribs and sternum in the way. Pulling hard on a retractor designed by an intern-hating pervert, I was suffering a hooked handle poking right into the soft spot between thumb and index finger. I was yanking it up and away from my body, while trying with the other hand to suck blood away, or hold the incision open. In a training program, there were often several bodies to do the pulling; and thirty years later there are ingenious erector-set devices to hold all sorts of retractors at once. On this occasion it was me and Lester. I'm sure he'd have been yelling at the poor exposure in another situation, but now he was all business, still silent. This went on for an hour or two, until it was clear we weren't going to find a specific source. "Damn"—barely audible— was about the only word he spoke from incision to closure.

The bail-out option is to cut the nerves to the stomach (a vagotomy). It can work by reducing acid production, and temporarily reducing blood flow to the area. There are two main vagus nerve trunks, running down the esophagus. To find them, you encircle the esophagus right where it joins the stomach and apply a little stretching, which makes the nerves tighten like guitar strings. In an open operation, reaching down, with lousy exposure, it can be made easier by slinging the esophagus with a long rubber ribbon (a Penrose drain) and tugging on it while feeling for the nerves. That requires passing an angled clamp behind the esophagus and over to the left, getting the drain into the teeth of the clamp, and pulling it back to the right. And so we did. As Lester felt around for the nerves, I watched his eyes as they squinted over his mask into the wound. Unable to see into the hole, I was trying to read progress in his face. I saw his pupils get big, his skin go fish-white, and his jaw tighten as he realized he'd passed the clamp not behind the esophagus, but through it. Harpooned. Silently, trembling from fingertip to shoulder, Lester sutured the two holes, thinking, I'm certain, that he'd killed the man. (The esophagus often heals poorly.) I struggled to hold the retractor in any way to help. A couple of drains were placed, in case of leakage, and then we beat a retreat.

The relative was now my charge. I kept track of his fluid needs, watched his vital signs, held his hand, carted him to X-ray, managed his tubes, hung more blood. Staying close for many days and nights, I gave graveyard-whistling encouragement to him and his fairly famous family. Dr. Weisman came and went, didn't say much. On morning rounds, I let the resident staff know what was going on. It was a long ride, and scary for a time, not looking good—fevers, more bleeding, too much drainage from the tubes. But eventually there was resolution, and the relative made it home, weak, thin, tired, and grateful to me for saving his life. His whole family told me that. Interesting. Clearly I hadn't saved his life, but by being there, being positive, cracking the occasional joke, and making it obvious that I was with him, they saw it that way. Noted.

Lester never said anything specific to me about it all, but when I'd see him in a hallway, he'd smile his ambiguous smile and sometimes he'd flap his hand my way. "Say, uh, Schwaaab . . . would you, uh . . . would you . . . like some . . . tickets to the . . . Forty-Niners game?"—reaching for his wallet and pawing inside. Once I sat in the surgery lounge as he ate a sack lunch, hunched over his little brown bag, nibbling on a sandwich held close, maybe trying to store it in his cheeks.

"Dr. Weisman, I see you have a white shoelace and a black one. Is that so you can tell left from right?"

"Yeah . . . the uh . . . white is . . . left. The uh . . . black . . . is . . . right."

"Gee, Dr. Weisman, it looks like it's just the opposite."

". . . huh huh huh huh huh . . ."

I know he wrote me a stellar recommendation for selection as a resident.

A few years later Lester Weisman died, and when he did I was asked to be a pallbearer at his funeral. I was seriously flattered. When I went by the surgery office to give my affirmation, I made the mistake of fishing: of course I will. Can you tell me why I was asked? Because you're big, and you're on Pathology so you have the time. Wear your whites.

UCSF is a referral center. Not a lot of simple cases, not many young healthy people. So the nurses were plainly thrilled when Gary Davis was admitted, a big blond surfer dude from Southern California. Handsome and gregarious, he was perfect nurse-bait except for the huge hard lump in his neck: his thyroid, which should have been soft and invisible. Clearly malignant. Why he came all that way to have Dr. Griswold operate remains a mystery, but there we were, in the OR, struggling to get that thing out of Gary's neck. Ordinary thyroid surgery is very tidy. The thyroid is like the trinket in a surprise package; you open one layer after another, each prettier than the last. Once there, if you get your finger in exactly the right place, not a filament too deep or shallow, you can sweep in front and behind each lobe of the gland, popping it forward and partly out of the neck. Because there's critical anatomy behind the gland, you have to contain your excitement. But the dissection is nevertheless a classic exercise in anatomy.

Except now. Besides being huge and stony, Gary's gland was stuck to everything, even the skin over it. It became obvious there was no way it was coming out. All that was possible was a biopsy to find out what type of cancer it was and, because his trachea was already distorted by the tumor, a tracheostomy to prevent future airway obstruction (placing a breathing tube directly into the trachea). "Trach," pronounced "trake," is the abbreviated term. Placing a trach tube is usually not difficult, especially with the neck wide open and absent a respiratory emergency. The normal thyroid drapes over the trachea but doesn't obscure it. In this case, however, it was necessary to chisel through rock to get there, and having finally exposed the trachea, no available tube was long enough or shaped appropriately to pass through this huge gland and angle comfortably into the trachea. Tracheostomy tubes are prefabricated, in various sizes, relatively soft plastic, but not customizable. So Gary left the OR with the longest tube we could find, precariously placed and barely reaching far enough. And I left feeling sick at the thought of this young guy facing a miserable death. Then, a couple of days later, as he returned from another trip to the OR to have placed a custom-made and fitted metal tube, we got the good news: his biopsy showed Hodgkin's disease rather than thyroid cancer. Radiation to his neck might cure him; he began treatment immediately.

Generously sharing my ever-increasing knowledge and confidence, I was making Sunday morning rounds with a medical student. Halfway through checking on a couple of dozen postops, we got to Gary. He was feeling good. Except that, he wrote, when he coughed he'd noticed a streak or two of blood. He showed me a tissue: barely a drop. Not a big deal, I figured; with a metal tube, a little irritation seemed perfectly expected. I told him I'd mention it to Dr. Griswold and not to worry about it, and we moved on to the remaining patients. A few minutes later, when I heard a nurse yelling, "There's someone bleeding in the shower!" Gary was the last person on my mind as I sprinted up the hall. I'd never heard of a tracheo-innominate fistula.

The innominate artery is about as big around as your little finger and arises from the arch of the aorta, which is the main artery leaving the heart. It supplies blood to the brain and the right arm, and it runs just in front of the trachea as the trachea bends backward and becomes the two main bronchi. A fistula is a connection between two hollow structures, or between a hollow structure and, say, the skin. Usually it suggests some bowel content leaking somewhere— an unpleasant problem but not an emergency. To call a connection between the trachea and the innominate artery a "fistula" seems like calling a plane crash an "aero-earth interface." But that's the official medical term. Tracheostomy tubes bend forward, necessary to pass through the skin and front wall of the trachea, and aim into the chest. It's not a problem, usually. The backward bend in the trachea is well below the end of the trach tube. But a low-placed (continued)

It was a cheap horror movie, switching from black and white to color at the scariest moment. I opened the shower door to see Gary wilting, collapsing slowly like a leaking balloon, melting onto the floor as pint after pint of blood sprayed from his neck with each cough, the white tile walls by now splashed fatally red. Momentarily paralyzed, I felt as if blood were draining from me as well. Somehow, I acted, and as we dragged Gary across the hall to his bed, I called for an IV set-up and managed to get a needle into a big vein. The blood bank was two floors below. Using the handrails like parallel bars, I swung over several stairs at a time, knocked open the lab door, demanded ten units of O-negative blood, STAT!! ("STAT" is the oft-used medical term for "right now!" Its origin is mysterious. O-negative blood is the "universal donor"; in a true emergency it's pretty safe to give it without knowing the recipient blood type. It has none of the proteins to which the body forms anti-blood antibodies, so reactions are rare, and mild.)

"Who's the patient? We need the ID card...." Calm and official.

"Goddamn it, he's dying, just give it to me!!" I was already clammy and scared to death.

Such a thing would likely never happen today, but the tech backpedaled into the lab and brought out a few bags of blood. I vaulted back up the stairs and squeezed as much blood as I could into the now-lifeless body of Gary Davis. We gave CPR and tried

---

(continued) tube, either by necessity (huge thyroid) or by error—and especially a metal one as opposed to the soft plastic ones with a pillow-like balloon at the end— can be rubbing on the front wall of the trachea. With time—made worse by inflammation from, say, radiation—such a tube can erode through the wall and into the artery. Disaster. And at that point in medical history, always fatal.

unsuccessfully to contact Dr. Griswold. Sunday morning at Moffitt Hospital, where emergencies didn't happen. Crushed, exhausted, and shaking, sitting on Gary's bed, I had no idea what just occurred, what more I could have done. The medical student stood there looking shocked; but, unlike me, he had the comfort of knowing he was off the hook. I wished he'd go away. When Griswold finally called in, he told me that if I'd informed him of the blood, he'd have taken Gary straight to the OR.

I couldn't stop thinking about it. Would that vision ever leave me? Should it? Gary coughing away his life in explosions of blood, me running toward him, weighted down.... I wondered if I should continue in surgery training and wasn't sure if I should even live. Ideally, a surgeon knows everything; realistically, he must at least know what he doesn't know. Is that even possible? I learned later that it is. A huge part of surgery training is incubating a sense of limits. Chain of command. Don't make decisions without checking up to the next level. You know nothing. If something goes wrong, it's because someone screwed up, probably you: and here's what you did wrong. As miserable as that can be, it's also vital. There's nothing more dangerous than a doctor who doesn't know when he has wandered outside his zone of competence. Of course, there are no perfectly infallible solutions to any situation. What we do is a sophisticated game of odds-playing. Given these data (which are usually incomplete and often conflicting) the odds are if we do this, that will happen. But maybe not. So at UCSF, at least with the best of the profs, the great sin was not to have a bad outcome. If a reasoned measure was taken of the important issues, and a careful, thoughtful decision made, then complications were not always criticized. Dissected, surely. Evaluated. Options reviewed. But heads might not roll. However, if an important issue was overlooked, or if a decision was carried out without proper following of chain of command, all hell would (rightfully) break loose.

Had a sympathetic and supportive chief resident not taken me aside the next day and assured me that there was no way Griswold would have done anything on the basis of a few streaks of blood, I'm pretty sure I'd have ended my training, one way or another. Having done dozens of tracheostomies over the years, I've finally let myself believe that the chief was right. (Not to mention the fact that had Griswold answered his phone—which he hadn't—and had he headed in immediately—which he didn't—Gary's artery would still have blown long before the doctor got there. The realization comes to me only now, as I write this book, and it eases, a bit.) I have seen blood streaks in mucus from a trach many a time since then. Always knowing that the tube was well-placed, and soft, I never felt the need to do anything about it. And never, after training, did I see another tracheo-innominate fistula. (Notice that I said "after training".)

There were other characters on the Blue Service. The busiest private surgeon, with good reason, Maurice Galante performed operations that moved smoothly and quickly, and his patients did well. He had an attractive Italian accent, which he used to good effect. (I believe he was born in the USA: I always wondered if he sounded like Brooklyn at home.) "Seed," he would say. "Let us make [r-rolling] rrounds." He'd written a text on breast cancer and was called occasionally to testify in court. A friend of mine was a malpractice attorney (defended doctors, obviously) and loved to use Maurice as a witness. Asked if he considered himself an expert, so my friend told me, Dr. Galante would say, "No one eez an experrt. But my own mahtherr had brreast cancer. . . ."

Once he was operating with a resident and they both leaned toward the incision at the same time, bumping heads. "Ah, Dr. Galante, a meeting of the minds." "Yez," he said. "And I feel so alone." He occasionally took me to lunch at one of his many favorite restaurants, where he'd be greeted as "Il doctore" and hustled to the best table. I hoped, as I watched others operate, that someday I'd be able to do it as well as Maurice Galante.

Then there was Howard O'Reilly. A wraith. Older than the buildings. Dressed in a starched and shiny white coat, he'd materialize pushing a cart of his special bandages, see his patients alone, shuffling down the hall like an ancient peddler: cotton for muscles, alive alive-o. He allowed no one, not even the nurses, to see what was going on under his dressings. Taking forever to operate, he'd spend hours just getting an incision made and adhesions divided, which made me think that if this is surgery, I want no part of it. He blinked a lot and never looked anyone in the eye. Denying such "modern" concepts as fluid management or measuring venous pressure, he provoked violent fantasies as he refused to listen to our concerns about his post-ops.

Normally the surfaces within the belly are shiny and slippery. After an operation, or subsequent to infection or injury, some of the shiny things adhere to each other: thus, adhesions. Depending on how extensive and how old (the older the less bloody, and therefore the easier) it can take a while to hack through them.

Track him down in the parking lot, we'd imagine. Kick him a few times. I thought it inexcusable that he remained on staff, well past his prime.

Internship is about osmosis: learning by absorption, by being there. There are no classes, no curriculum, no exams. It's the ultimate descendant of apprenticeship—highly-caffeinated, on-the-job training. Learning derives from seeing and doing, and from randomly strewn pearls of wisdom, tossed to you when appropriate to the moment. On the Blue Service, I began to have an understanding of the process. You provide enormous amounts of work to many people who, in return, give you the occasional particle of knowledge. See enough post-op patients, and you start to get a sense of what's normal and what's not. What happens to urine output, how much IV fluid is right, what works best for pain. Call the attending often enough, and you learn what information is needed to make an assessment. Post-op fever? How's the wound, the lungs, the urine? Make 'em get up, walk, cough. Pulse going up? Your mind begins to produce a list of causes, of actions. A cancer patient here, a person with gallstones there; fragments of understanding break off and re-form in your mind, puzzle pieces to be put together while you're not looking. In the operating room, even at the far end of the table, you can hear whispers from your future. Lessons get learned, whether you know it or not. It's a wishful proposition, like mama playing Mozart to the baby in her womb.

four

A Little Girl and Her Kidneys

"It's never this busy; it's gonna slow down." I heard that every day I was on the Transplant Service. Kidneys, and the people who needed them, kept showing up, needing attention whether or not there was time or room. Killer. In the 1970s, more kidney transplants were done at UCSF than anywhere else in the world. The two main men were Sam Kountz, one of the few black surgeons in high places in academia, and Fred Belzer, who had perfected the first machine to keep a kidney alive after removing it from a donor. Coincidentally, this machine was known as the Belzer.

It was a huge thing at that time: prior to its invention, a kidney removed from a cadaver donor was flushed, packed in ice, and taken to the recipient hospital where it needed to be implanted within hours. That could mean, in some cases, a wasted kidney if a suitable recipient wasn't immediately available, or placing it when it was beginning to deteriorate. There was a window of only a few hours. The Belzer, with its pulsatile flow and special solution pumping through the kidney, opened that window to two or three days.

Dr. Belzer had a faint Germanic accent, wavy hair, and a

singer's baritone voice—TV doc quality, had he so chosen. Dr. Kountz was, I thought, notably comfortable in his uniqueness as a black man on an otherwise nearly sheet-white staff. At a time when it seemed African-Americans in such places often felt the need to bleach their behavior, he didn't. He was a gifted surgeon and a straight-talk guy with a musical Southern accent. Seeing him in their rooms for only a minute at a time, patients nevertheless revered him. Once I assisted him in removing a hopelessly diseased, chronically infected, and huge cystic kidney, as was done before a transplant to avoid overwhelming infection. It was a difficult, bloody, and nearly impossible operation. Dr. Kountz was sweating, dripping into the wound. When he finally got the kidney out and controlled all the bleeding, he looked up at me and said, laughing and faking a new accent, "I ain't gonna do DAT no mo!" Dr. Kountz died several years ago of hypertensive crisis (wherein the blood pressure rises rapidly and disastrously). Rumor had it that when he arrived semi-comatose in a small hospital somewhere in New York, it was assumed that because he was black it was a drug OD, or drunkenness, and that by the time he got proper attention his brain was irreversibly damaged. I don't know it to be true. In any case, it was the premature loss of a great and gifted surgical leader.

Even with the Belzer machine, there was no time to lose when a kidney showed up. The pump allowed them to be brought in from further away, but when a match was made it was still a frenzy to get the recipient admitted and ready, and transplants were begun at whatever hour of day or night things fell into place. Night, usually. The operation itself tends to be easy, barring problems with the way the kidney was harvested (yes, that is the term: harvested), or with the target vessels of the patient. A kidney fits nicely just above the groin, hitching a ride on the artery and vein to the leg. In a slick trick, the ureter (the conduit of urine out of the kidney) gets tunneled through the muscle wall and sewn to the inside of the bladder. And then, in most cases, the patient starts peeing like crazy. Sometimes too crazy: a shocked kidney can make urine but it may be more like water than the real thing, and without care the patient can become severely dehydrated. Post-op care was the point of it all; the operation was nothing.

In those days, transplant rejection—an immune reaction—was managed by huge doses of steroids and other dangerous drugs, which indiscriminately suppressed all immunity. So when we weren't treating rejection, we were managing horrendous infections, of a sort not seen anywhere else in modern Western medicine: fungal infections of the sinuses, growing straight into the brain; yeast infections of the spinal cord; rare forms of pneumonia that made lungs look—and function—like cheap foam rubber. Nasty stuff. Signs of rejection led to ever higher doses of anti-rejection drugs. Amazingly, it took several years of watching patients die of infection for the light-bulb to blink on: it's better to save the patient than the kidney. If a doubling of the drug doses didn't reverse the rejection episode, it was time to stop the drugs and get the kidney the hell out of there.

I don't think even the higher-ups would deny that interns on the Transplant Service were little more than cheap round-the-clock laborers whose education was irrelevant. Kidney function and failure, ok, I learned a few things about that; but I really never needed to know how to treat mucormycosis (the fungus thing). With a ward full of transplanted patients, there were reams of lab data that needed tracking down and posting on a flow sheet for afternoon rounds, at which time Dr. Kountz or Belzer would briefly check the patient, look at the latest lab numbers, and announce the daily dose of whatever meds were to be given. I would have spent at least the prior hour or two in the lab, cajoling and sweet-talking the lab techs to help me find the data. We interns hustled every day to the lab, spent time copying the numbers onto the flow sheets outside each patient door, then stood deferentially aside while the masters made their pronouncements. For this I went to medical school? If results were missing, we heard about it. When we'd manage to scrounge a full complement for each patient, we might be graced with a nod that acknowledged our existence. Teaching was, mostly, not in their lexicon. More than anywhere else in the training process, I simply did the work I was given, made no decisions, had no input, did nothing for the patients that couldn't have been done by about five good servants, each working an eight-hour day. Well, except for Katy.

There aren't a lot of kids with kidney failure. Katy Dawkins was beautiful, very sick, and very scared, admitted to a service that could be cold and hurried. When she arrived, I was smitten and never entertained for a moment maintaining professional distance from this speed-talking, pig-tailed ten-year-old, freckled like a crumpet. Having had some unusual problems with matching, she was getting a kidney from her dad—and even he was much less than an ideal match. Such "living related" transplants were uncommon then, and she and her dad were admitted a few days early for preparations. That meant I had time to get to know Katy and her family. Dad was a big guy and seemed perfectly comfortable with the plan; he'd apparently already donated a bunch of his freckles. I liked to visit Katy at night, when no one else was around, and when I could usually spare a few minutes. We'd talk about the operation, or whatever else she had on her mind. Exchange corny jokes. She asked a little about me, too, and wanted to be sure I'd be in the operating room with her.

We were in side-by-side operating rooms. Dr. Kountz and Tony E., the resident, were with Katy, readying the field for the kidney. Dr. Belzer and I were with her dad, harvesting. Because Belzer still had work to do after the kidney was out, I was the one to carry it next door. A kidney is slippery as a fish in the grip of latex surgical gloves, so I had white cotton gloves over the rubber ones, for traction. Walking white-gloved into the next room, carrying a kidney, I felt as if I were somewhere between Jeeves and Jesus. With all eyes on me (did they wonder if I'd trip; could I do something horrible?), a nurse holding the door open as I walked in, I opted for concentration over contemplation. As I laid the kidney in a pan on the instrument table, I realized that I'd barely breathed on the walk from room to room, and that my hands were trembling. After going back and helping Dr. Belzer finish, I returned to watch the implantation. The kidney looked huge lying on Katy's belly. It seemed impossible to fit it in; shoehorned, it would pooch out like a tumor under her party dress, I guessed. I needn't have worried.

Hyperacute rejection is a hideous crime. The body, lurking in a dark alley until its victim wanders by, jumps the transplanted organ and, with unfeeling brutality and evil purpose, beats on it with everything it has, the unfairest of fights. There's no drug that can stop it. It was over in twenty-four hours. Swollen nearly to the point of splitting open, Dad's kidney ended up back in a pan—black, useless, killed.

Her dad was merely sad, disappointed, and sore. Katy was devastated; surely it was somehow her fault. As he hobbled toward her bed after a ride to her floor, she had a hard time looking at him. He, of course, told her it was ok, he was fine, it was just a bad thing that happened for no reason. She smiled and said she knew that, but at night when I visited her she sobbed from somewhere I couldn't reach, for herself, for her dad, for the reappearance of the dialysis machine (the artifical kidney, tethered to her for several hours a day, three or so days a week). I sat, listened, and gave her my hand. And then, a couple of days later, when she was about ready for discharge, a perverse and ironic miracle: a well-matching cadaver kidney appeared. I heard about it when I was in the OR with a routine transplant; as soon as I was free I raced to Katy's room and in front of her family and nurses, abandoning any pretense of decorum, I gave her a big hug and got back a happy kiss. The second transplant and recovery were routine: a minor rejection episode, a few days in the hospital, and home she went, peeing prettily. I saw her only once in the clinic before I went off the service, and she continued to do great.

Katy and I exchanged letters while I spent the next year in Vietnam. When I resumed training, among the first things on my list was to find out when she would be in clinic, to surprise her. The surprise was mutual. Two years of high-dose prednisone had accomplished the second perverse miracle: keep a kidney, lose your childhood. Body-snatched by a sexless troll, the beautiful girl was now unrecognizable: dwarfed and dystrophic, moon-faced and buffalo-humped. I know I failed to conceal my shock, and she her embarrassment. What, in God's name, had we accomplished? Would she have been better served by staying on dialysis until she'd grown more? Would she have survived that long? Was she a worthy sacrifice to our understanding, born too soon on the time line of medical progress? Is she still alive? I don't know the answer to any of those questions. I do know that, motivated by the obvious shortcomings of such treatments, new management and new drugs have been developed such that she'd have a nearly normal childhood and adulthood were she to reappear today. And that for the rest of my career, I've made myself and my patients think long and hard when embarking on a path whose downside and upside were nearly in balance.

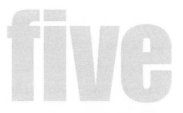

The Mission—Nearly Impossible

San Francisco General Hospital, "the County," was the essence of our surgical training, the crucible and the soul. More dignified and in some way predictable, the UCSF hospital—Moffit Hospital—was the medical center, the research hospital, where I'd started. The County was drama, fear, chaos, and excitement, the prism through which you saw yourself and your readiness to be a surgeon. A classic county hospital, decades old, it was made of solid brick, with incongruous fancy filigree—artsy details along the roof line, marble in the entryway—overlooked and no longer relevant to the seething survival-struggle that the place had come to embody. Slung low, with long hallways, too few and too slow elevators, SFGH housed patients in open wards, dank and under-lit warehouses, except for the rare private room used for people with dangerous infections, or for the occasional muckamuck waiting to get well enough to transfer the hell out of there. The County was, in a word, alive.

It also had a dark side, buried deep. Connecting the main building to the psych ward across the alley were long and claustrophobic tunnels—dangerous at any time for a lone woman, eerie even for me when I made the rare trip over there. Not sated by its diet of damaged people, the County sometimes coughed up its own cud from down there; assaults on employees, though uncommon, were not rare. But from a physician in training, and most especially from a surgeon, San Francisco General Hospital demanded love and got it easily, unconditionally. It's where I always wanted to be.

Located at the north end of the hospital, which was situated in San Francisco's Mission District, the emergency room was officially titled "Mission Emergency Hospital." We called it the Mission, or "the Mish." The staff at SFGH constituted a brew of the overworked and underpaid, speaking any of several languages. County employees drifted in various stages of burnout or apathy amongst a core of nurses, techs, and aides who were deeply dedicated, highly skilled, admirable beyond words.

There was an enlightened policy in San Francisco: all trauma cases—gunshots, jumpers, stab wounds, accident victims, cops and criminals and innocent bystanders—and most other emergency patients were swept up and brought to the Mission by county-run ambulances. And come they did, in an unsteady stream, day and night. The many private hospitals were out of the picture. One of a handful of true trauma centers in the country at that time, SFGH rightly had a reputation as one of the best, largely because of one man— F. William Blaisdell, "the Blazer." They say ontogeny repeats phylogeny; phys-

There was a brief throwback: bowing to political pressures and the misguided beliefs of some hospitals that they should have some of the action, the city for a time lifted the rules and made it a come-one, come-all race to the scene, with the winning ambulance getting the choice of where to go. It took only a couple of disasters—people dying for lack of basic trauma services—before it reverted back to common sense. Whatever else it was or wasn't, the County was where you wanted to be in a crunch.

iognomy follows its own rules. Blazer looked sweetly benign: glasses, rosy cheeks, a bit soft. Nice smile, natty bow tie. Nerdish, even. A math teacher, a pussycat. Well, not exactly. To cross the Blazer was to exit training, naked. He was Chief of Surgery at the County, and trauma was his baby. He'd set up the rules. There was accountability from top to bottom and back to top. Two trauma teams were led by a single chief resident, who lived in the hospital for his two-month stint, present every hour, non-stop. Below the chief were two senior residents, who led each of the two teams, alternating 24-hour shifts (often more like 30 or 36 hours). In addition to the senior residents, there were junior residents, a couple of interns, and several students. Separate interns and residents, medical and surgical, worked full-time in the emergency room.

When a trauma case arrived, the trauma team was called, but the initial care was begun by the ER-based surgical members. Trauma rooms in the ER were kept at the ready, with IVs connected to tubing ready to go, various instrument packs cooked and available. An OR was free at all times, with staff. When necessary, a trauma patient could be wheeled into the trauma room, get tubes placed in various orifices or in holes we made, IVs going, blood started, necessary X-rays done, and be up in an OR with all personnel ready to cut, in about ten minutes. It wasn't pretty; the Mission was not designed with such a drill in mind. Wheeled through doors used by all, the victims went down a hall crammed with people of all ages and any of several sexes awaiting help with all manner of maladies, into the trauma room. After resuscitation, they'd be brought back out, down the same hall, maybe with a stop in X-ray, then into another and bigger hall, past more people, to an elevator theoretically dedicated to trauma cases but which might instead be transporting janitors, visitors, or crazies, in colorful combinations. The elevator was way too slow and too small, but it served—especially if a med student had been sent ahead of the gurney to call for and evacuate the thing in time.

Once, when I was chief resident, we had a typical extravaganza: gunshot wound requiring opening the chest in the ER, clamping the aorta, giving direct heart massage. The victim's family had descended on the place and was massed outside the trauma room, at least twenty of them. A path was cleared as we made our way to the elevator, I with my hand in his chest, squeezing the heart, bloody and proud. Stand back, let us through. Elevator door barely able to close as the family leaned in en masse. Let us do our job, we'll take care of him. Doors finally shut, and the elevator goes . . . down. The OR is up. A couple of janitors had finished their smokes and had called the elevator to take them back up, against the "rules." So, moments after closing, the family sees the elevator doors reopen, revealing the scene just witnessed: family outside, us inside, me squeezing the heart. Let us do our job, we'll take care of him. . . .

The attending surgeons at the County all took turns covering trauma, and when they did, they were expected to work nearly as hard as the residents, which meant being available at all times of day or night to consult, to come to the OR. But Blazer himself was the overlord and reserved the right to stick his fingers in at any time. And there were certain rules. One, we never wore scrubs (the pajamas you see surgical types wearing) except in the OR. In patient care areas, we wore our whites and dress shirts, and at all times a necktie. No beards. Business cards with our names and numbers were given to every patient we saw. Drunks, derelicts, addicts—all were expected to be treated respectfully. And I learned why, having seen the look in the eyes of a heart-attack victim as I, in my white coat and tie, handed him off to the coronary care resident: the resident with his long hair, scraggly beard, a wrinkled and dirty lab coat covered with happy-face and peace buttons. Fear is what I saw. But Blazer could take it too far; I watched an intern present a patient to him, the man hanging on after hours of surgery done to put together pieces of his insides rended apart by a MUNI bus (San Francisco's municipal bus service). The intern was proud of his care, detailing a night of work which had begun the moment the operation ended and continued non-stop until morning. Blazer interrupted, saying, "I can't hear a word you're saying, mister. All I can see is that you're not wearing a tie."

Dr. Blaisdell was more concerned about process than outcome; actions taken had to be based on thorough and thoughtful consideration of all the possibilities, after having been properly vetted at the next level. Do that, have a bad result, and he'd back you up. Fail to think a thing through, overlook something, don't follow the chain of command—even though with trauma the time frame could be nano-seconds—you'd best prepare for a memorable reckoning. A fellow resident, now a respected academic surgeon, once performed an emergency tracheostomy in the ER on a man turning blue. This was prior to the invention of the Heimlich maneuver; the man was choking on food. Richard swept his finger through the patient's mouth and throat, dislodging nothing, and decided a trach was needed. Which he did, finding the chunk of meat in the guy's mouth after the man pinked up. Too quick on the trigger? Maybe. But in deciding to do the trach, the sin was that when the nurse asked if she should call the trauma team, Rich said no, he could handle it. Next day, Dr. Blaisdell called him in. Deeply shaken, Rich later recounted the story. No words were spoken except these: "A cat has nine lives. A surgical resident has two. You've used one. Now get out of my office."

My first experience at the County was in the Mission, where I was one of many interns from surgery, medicine, family practice, responsible for whatever problems presented. I started on the evening shift. The door to the trauma room was open when I arrived, and a brief glance inward was enough to reveal everything I needed to know: the place seemed to shimmer with the dying heat of a failed trauma rescue. Partially covered, the victim was still there, his disconnected breathing tube having funnelled his last breath upward. There were tubes in each side of his chest, attached to plastic receptacles, the collection chambers of which were filled with blood, while the water-seal chambers—because they were still attached to suction—sighed soothing polyrhythmic burbles. (People in nice homes pay good money for fountains to make those sounds outside their bedroom windows.) Splashed on the open instrument packs and pooled on the floor was the man's blood; and on the sheets, and on his one visible hand, hanging relaxed under a side-rail. IV bottles dangled with tubes attached, the fluids turned off. Hooked to the side of the gurney, the bag at the end of his bladder catheter held bright yellow and healthy-looking urine, probably still warm, attesting like a mood ring to his just-passed normality. Soon he'd be covered with a fresh sheet, the gurney piloted out, its wobbly wheel painting a sanguineous serpentine stripe part-way to the door. Efficient, talking about the trivia of life, a couple of people would mop up, disinfect, hang new tubes from fresh bottles, and lay out fresh instrument packs, making ready for the next victim to enter with fresh hope, like the happy couple shown to their crisp and perfumed honeymoon suite, carefully deceived and deliberately unmindful of the sweaty and fluid-soaked tryst played out on their very bed the night before. (Would you go in there if you knew?)

When an ambulance called in with a trauma victim on the way, I was expected to hustle to the trauma room. Otherwise, I stayed put and dealt with all comers: belly aches, headaches, drug ODs, pelvic infections, sore throats. Fractures and lacerations. Mission Emergency was the primary care center for thousands of dispossessed, depressed, and desperate people. Varying randomly among day, swing, and night shifts, we left our body clocks on the bedside table at home and worked twelve hours at a time, zombified within a couple of days. Some shifts we'd work up front in the initial contact and triage area, treating, suturing, sifting. Other days it was either the male or female holding rooms, to which patients were sent while awaiting tests, needing further observation before deciding disposition, waiting for any of the various specialty residents to come down to consult or admit them. Always there was tension between doing the best for the most people versus the best for the individual. With dozens of patients waiting to be seen, we knew there could be a serious illness ticking away while we were otherwise occupied. At first I took the time to connect every drunk with detox, extracting a promise to show up, or to get a social worker to see a homeless person, while more people piled up in the waiting areas, in the halls, on gurneys—some bleeding obsequiously, others raging, needing cops, needing the padded room (it was used to great advantage, every night). The triage system often being overwhelmed, we'd patrol the halls regularly, checking the parallel-parked gurneys for signs of life. We did many of the lab tests ourselves. Spin the blood in a centrifuge and check the red-cell level; make a smear of the blood and count the number and type of white cells. Spin the urine and check for various signs of trouble. It took up our time, but in the long run it was much faster than sending it to the lab and waiting for results.

It didn't take much soul-searching, or more than a few dressings-down by the senior folk, for me to realize the need for maximum efficiency: take the pie from the sky, put it where it could be consumed. If a drunk came in figuring he'd get a bed by saying he'd vomited blood and there was no evidence of it, we'd pass a tube into the stomach: if there was no blood, we'd poke a finger up the rear, testing the stool for blood. If there was still none, we'd check a blood count and if it was in a reasonable range, that was it—back out the door.

Headache: find out the history, check the vital signs, do a neurological exam, maybe make an appointment for the medical or neurology clinic, say goodbye. There was no choice. When it wasn't obvious that patients could safely be sent back out, they went to the holding ward for further evaluation and observation. On the night shift, the goal was to have the holding rooms empty by morning: not to have done so was proof to the trauma team, as they swept through in the morning to see the residue, that you'd failed in your job. Why is this person still here? What's the plan? When especially unsuccessful and exhausted, drained of empathy, I imagined hooking up hydraulics that would tilt the whole ward up at five a.m., back wall swinging outward, gurneys whooshing into a waiting dumpster.

It was in the female holding ward that I met Esther. A regular, she'd sometimes come in on her own, complaining of a belly ache; or she'd be brought in by ambulance, for an overdose or having been beaten up. Our first meeting was for abdominal pain, and as with every other woman having that complaint, the evaluation began with a pelvic exam, expecting pelvic inflammatory disease (PID): gonorrhea, mostly. The nurse had already put Esther up in stirrups when I met her. I said hello, asked a couple of questions, noted her quite attractive body, breasts barely covered by the gown (was that chest hair?). So it was not without surprise, as I settled in to do the pelvic exam, that I gazed upon the full complement of male paraphernalia. (Of course the nurse knew. It was the new-guy initiation.) She'd run out of money, or perhaps conviction, after undergoing breast implants and starting hormone treatments on her way to changing sexes. She really was a sad mess; her overdoses usually consisted of taking a homeopathic dose of something or other, then lying on a sidewalk where she'd be seen. Her assault visits followed picking up a guy and not explaining herself in a timely manner. I suppose she got more love (or was it condescension?) in the ER than anywhere else; over the course of many years all the nurses, interns, and residents got to know her well, and to notice her absence when she'd be gone for a few weeks, admitted to a mental hospital somewhere up the valley. When Esther stopped showing up, the rumor was she'd finally taken a dose of the real thing.

The ER surgical resident was in charge of the trauma room until the trauma team arrived, and he or she would assign duties. I liked to do cutdowns. No matter how deflated a victim's blood volume might be, the saphenous vein could be accessed, by virtue of its large size and predictable location, just in front of the inside of the ankle. Throw on a little iodine, a little local anesthetic if the patient was wide awake, make a transverse half-inch cut. A couple of tricks with a small curved clamp and an eleven blade (shaped like a tall right triangle: the cutting edge is on the angled side, and comes to a sharp point), and you're ready to insert a tube large enough to handle high-volume fluids. Could be done in less than a minute, not counting the time I'd spend looking up at the resident and waiting for a smile of approval.

CAT scans (fancy X-rays that give a good picture of the internal organs and their surrounds) are pretty routine now, but early in my training they were unavailable, and when they first appeared they were limited by their slowness. So we had other methods of assessment. Like taking a trip to the OR. Any penetrating injury—stab, gunshot, impalement—nearly without exception went for exploratory surgery: a quick squirt of dye and an overhead X-ray to see if there were two working kidneys, then up and away. Better, Dr. Blaisdell said, to take a look than to miss something serious. Given the state of imaging art, it made sense in the '70s; but the "negative lap" ("lap" is short for laparotomy, or opening the abdomen) was pretty common, meaning we often opened someone up and found nothing. For reasons unknown to me, a negative lap was called a "white owl," and there was a statue of one in the OR, the stuff nightmares are made of. Many were the times, over the years, that I closed an incision while a nurse held up the plaster owl, grinning, no doubt, behind her mask. Sometimes the whole crew would chant "white owl, white owl," like the opposing crowd at a basketball game, relishing an air-ball.

For blunt trauma, the need for exploration might or might not be obvious: a distended, tender belly along with unstable blood pressure meant there was surely something bad enough happening to warrant surgery. In a more subtle situation, we often did a peridial (short for "peritoneal dialysis")—putting a tube through the abdominal wall in amongst the viscera, infusing a liter of saline, and drawing it back to look for blood. Doing a peridial was about the most critical and invasive thing an ER intern could do in the trauma room (in fact it was usually done by the resident), and it made me nervous: it's possible to poke a hole in the bowel or vessels, or to fail to get the tube in the proper layer and get a false reading by putting the fluid outside the abdominal cavity. I did hear once from the trauma team that they found a hole in the bowel, before I got the hang of it. I wondered what would have happened had I poked the bowel when the peridial didn't trigger a lap. As a resident, I did plenty of peridials, never again, as far as I know, puncturing anything.

How much intervention should be done by the medics at the scene of the injury? Since San Francisco is a compact area, and given its well-organized trauma care system, the concept was "scoop and run." Get the patient in the ambulance and to the ER as fast as possible. The delay from starting an IV in the field can lead to more loss of blood volume than would have been replaced by the time the IV and fluid got in on the street. So the medics, while very skilled at what they did, were not always attentive to field-diagnosis. Once we responded to the trauma room to prepare for someone coming in "code three" (lights flashing, sirens blaring) with "exsanguination and evisceration" (massive bleeding and guts hanging out). I was puzzled to hear the patient talking and laughing as she rode the gurney into the room. Turns out she'd had several operations in the past, with complications that eventually made it impossible to close her abdominal wall. So she'd had skin grafts laid directly onto her intestines. It held her together just fine, but to look at her belly was to see the outline of her intestines worming around under the thin grafts. Now she'd scraped her belly, smaller than a skinned knee, and someone had evidently panicked. As the eight or ten people in the room faded away to where they were needed, I placed a bandaid and sent her on her way. (It occurs to me now; maybe the medics were just jerking our chain.)

On another occasion, when the medics called in multiple victims with gunshot wounds to the head, I made my way to the trauma room expecting bits of brain on blankets—something I've never gotten used to. With the sirens winding down, I saw two gurneys wheeled side by side toward us. Why were the women screaming and flailing at each other? Because the weapon involved had been a .22 pistol, fired by one at the other's head, after which the second lady grabbed the gun and shot back, into the face of number one. They'd been fighting over their mutual boyfriend, a cop we knew from the ER, who'd been the one to call it in. We started some IVs but restrained ourselves from the full drill. Despite a hole in one lady's forehead, and one in the other's cheek, neither had any signs of significant damage. On X-ray, the first had a bullet nicely smashed against an otherwise intact skull. The X-ray of the second showed . . . nothing. Interesting: a bullet hole in the face and no sign of a fragment anywhere in the head. Then a flash: take an X-ray of her belly. And there it was in her stomach. Entering the sinus in her cheek, the bullet had passed into the back of her throat, and she'd swallowed it. Cute. A prescription for antibiotics, and she was back to the shooting gallery. We expected at least one of them to be wheeled back to us in a few days, but I guess they settled it in other ways.

Drug overdoses came in around the clock—grizzled old guys, men and women who looked three times their age, and kids way too young. After resuscitation, they were all admitted, all given tickets to rehab. But most were lost forever, usually to heroin.

Treating overdoses was my first experience with a miracle drug: squirt some Narcan into the vein of an unconscious addict, and within seconds he or she went from comatose to awake, screaming and clawing their way back from pin-point pupils, blue skin, and vomit all over their clothes. (Narcan is short for "narcotic antagonist." Those really were the good old days: drug names made sense.) Starting an IV was the trick: usually the addict had long-since destroyed his veins, leaving scars and abscesses in their place. He might be down to using the underside of his tongue, or the dorsal vein of the penis. (Women run out of options sooner.) But none could ruin my personal domain, the saphenous vein. No one can get along without a surgeon.

The Mission gaveth, and tooketh away. Handling scores of patients a day, you gain skills and confidence, and lose little bits of humanity. Every patient who came was in need. Too broke, too drunk, too addicted, too crazy, most were there because they had no other choice. You'd think trauma, at least, would be an equal-opportunity calamity. But we had a saying, a truism: trauma happens to people who are asking for it. (The corollary: survival of trauma is inversely related to one's value to society.) Such rules are pretty much limited to trauma centers in large country hospitals—I'll give you that. Yet compassion itself can become a victim after getting spit at, sworn at, lunged at by the people we were trying to help. I watched in admiration as a bearded (and therefore compassionate) family practice intern struggled to hold still the head of a gunshot victim who was thrashing and swearing, resisting despite his severe wound. The man managed to twist his head around and bite the thumb of the intern, whose immediate response was to shout, "YOU BIT ME!" and pull his hand back into a fist, ready to strike. But showing amazing control and taking a deep breath, he stepped away and walked into the hall, where I saw him pace up and down, talking to himself. Finally, after a minute or two of deep reflection and meditative self-analysis, he strode back to the head of the stretcher and looked down at the guy, thoughtful and calm. And popped him one in the nose.

As an ER intern, trauma was exciting and fun; it punctuated long days with drama and a sense of accomplishment (and with a chance to admire the trauma team in action). But the responsibility was minimal, the duties almost rote. We were in the business of stabilization and intubation, making ready for surgery, then handing the patient off to the trauma team. Deciding what to do, repairing devastation, caring for the after-effects—that's where the action really was, as well as the pressure, the danger, and the real rewards. That came much later.

SIX

On to Vascular Surgery

The vascular surgery department at the UCSF hospital was a kingdom unto itself, ruled by Jack Wylie, who though less known to the general public, was, in the history of vascular surgery, an originator akin to Michael Debakey. At his side, in an uneasy alliance, jockeying for the future crown, were Steve Lefkowitz and Ken Rockford. They couldn't have been more different: Wylie the gruff, the taciturn, the steady. Harrumphed a lot, had a rarely seen but sharp sense of humor. Operating with him was always daunting because of his simmering fearsomeness, but often it was sprinkled with bits of information and occasional actual teaching. He was missing part of his right index finger, yanked away by a rope on his sailboat.

Smooth and elegant, Lefkowitz was comfortable and magnanimous in his wealth, handsome, well-dressed. Not really interested in the professorial aspects of being at a university hospital, he had a nice practice sprinkled with the rich and known, could do without a lot of teaching—at least of interns and junior residents—and wasn't interested in research. Of the three, Lefkowitz was the most predictably nice guy. Fun to operate with, free with jokes and pleasant topical intraoperative conversation.

Ken Rockford was a goddamn grenade. Intense, wound-up, possessed by a temper that could induce self-soilage by those in the blast zone, he was also the most gifted surgeon, and a restless innovator. Wylie hadn't exactly rested on his laurels, and he was interested in and encouraging of the cutting-edge work Rockford did, but was not so much out in front anymore. Ken Rockford always had ideas, developed new techniques, took on the most difficult cases. When things were going well, he could be a brilliant teacher, pleasant and approachable. When not, he might lash out in the most vicious and hurtful ways: squinting and snarling, insulting and threatening. And once in a while, he'd pop for no damn reason at all. Because the vascular department brought in lots of patients and money, and had a national reputation for excellence, the triumvirate had power unequaled by any other department. They knew that no one would call them to heel, and they acted like it. They ran their department as they saw fit, and were left alone to do so.

While the political subtleties might not have been apparent to us interns, we knew well in advance that working on the vascular service would be a grueling trial. Sick people, and lots of them: all three surgeons admitted several a day and had little sympathy for an intern's travails. Vascular patients, as a rule, are elderly, have accompanying heart disease, hypertension, often diabetes. The operations are high risk. Emergencies happen: a ruptured aneurysm (a weakening and dilatation of an artery—usually the abdominal aorta, the largest artery in the body), threatening and often accomplishing loss of life; an occluded vessel to the leg, ready to cause loss of limb; a carotid artery firing off warning shots to the brain. You might be in the operating room for many hours on a single case, with others left to go, and patients piling up on the floors waiting for pre-op workup, or post-op care. Some bled post-op; some had strokes or heart attacks. All required intensive care for a while: careful fluid management, watching the kidneys, keeping track of the blood sugar, checking pulses and hollering if they disappeared. Pushing the limits of the possible, it was a one-intern service; nights were frequently without sleep. Catnaps when a moment presented itself were a necessity.

Other than the fact that the only time to get to it might be two a.m, admitting patients became routine: take a history, do an exam, get a permit, draw blood. All abdominal cases got a cut-down in an arm vein, against the need to infuse large volumes of blood or fluid in the OR. We took and read our own EKGs. On one occasion, the tracing on one of Dr. Wylie's big cases looked a little scary, and I called him about it. "Hmph. We're not operating on the heart, doc." End of discussion.

This was my first service on which there was a chief resident who loomed large. (There was a chief on Blue, but he spent most of his time wishing he had more to do.) The vascular clinic produced "staff" patients, most of whom would be operated on by the chief. In fact, given the volume of the vascular program, chief residents might finish the UCSF program having fixed more aneurysms than hernias. (Vascular surgery now is done mostly by general surgeons who've completed an additional fellowship; chief residents don't do as much of it anymore.) In addition to letting the chief work on clinic patients, Doctors Wylie/Lefkowitz/Rockford ceded most of the post-op care of their own patients to the resident staff, knowing there was always an uptight chief in charge who'd hear about it if care were less than excellent. Embodying the layperson's stereotypical view of a surgeon, the chief resident while I was rotating through was John Haugen: tough-looking, loud, certain about the rightness of everything he did, and anxious to share that certainty with anyone in shouting distance. He was demanding, but he worked his own butt off, was fair, and a damn good surgeon. Hidden deep in his thrust-out chest, below his equally thrust-out chin, was a kind heart. Once or twice, after a particularly exhausting stretch of work and, I assume, what he considered good effort and results, he'd demand I go home, saying he'd cover for me. I do mean demand; there was no saying "no" to John, even if you were a patient.

Harvey Ashcroft was a miserable wreck of a guy, admitted to the vascular service for a last-ditch effort to save his legs. He'd had every possible operation on every possible blood vessel in his body. Take away the cholesterol deposits and there'd be nobody left in his bed. His legs were purple and mottled, as the few blood cells who'd made it down there staggered away, depleted of all their oxygen, heading for another circuit through his barely beating heart and water-logged lungs, getting re-loaded with a few molecules of oxygen, then forced once again into a fruitless attempt to make it to his toes. Giving up as well, Harvey's weakened heart muscles had stretched thin and dilated until the heart filled his chest, barely squeezing, and doing it so pitifully slowly that he was on pills to try to make it beat faster. He'd had all the bypasses, all the ream-jobs that were possible. Now he was in for a sympathectomy (oh, the irony), in which nerves that control muscles within the blood vessels (called the sympathetic nerves) are cut, in hopes of relaxing the vessels and increasing flow. In Harvey's case, the vessels were lead pipes filled with sludge; not much chance of working, but it's all there was, and he was a persuasive guy. After the operation, through which he miraculously lived, and seeing that it did no good whatsoever, he talked his cardiologist into trying a pacemaker, hoping that further cranking up his heart rate would improve circulation. He remained persuasive. A temporary pacemaker was placed, tuned to about seventy beats, as opposed to his drug-flogged fifty, and Harvey went into worse heart failure.

Stoking ourselves during an atypical lull, John and I were sitting in the cafeteria one Saturday morning when the operator paged overhead, "Dr. Schwab, 7A, STAT." The vascular floor. I made toward the four flights of stairs. "NO, Sidney! NEVER run up the stairs!! Take the elevator so you're not out of breath when you get there." (John had lots of rules.) We arrived to find Mr. Ashcroft in the tiny treatment room, wheeled there, bed and all, by the nurses. He thrashed about, angrily producing invective, while we learned the story: somehow he'd secreted a gun in his luggage, planning his own solution if none of his operations worked. He'd fired a round at his chest, aiming for his heart but missing, despite the fact that it was the size of a volleyball. A tidy little hole with a gunpowder ring around it, at the bottom of his left ribcage, testified to the seriousness of his intent. "Let me die, let me die, damn you all!" Harvey Ashcroft cried. John Haugen grabbed a fistful of gown and lifted him off his bed, shaking the frail and withering torso, leaning his face down into Harvey's, trading flecks of spittle. "Goddamn it, Mr. Ashcroft, you're not dying on MY service, you sonofabitch." Off to the OR we went, the trauma nerves in John's brain firing twenty-one-gun volleys. Sliced him open snick-snick (remarkable in itself for a Saturday at Moffitt), to find his spleen lying there in two pieces, neatly cut in half by the bullet. If you had done that to yourself, by now there'd be several pints of blood filling the field. In Mr. Ashcroft's case, given the pathetic output of his heart, there were about two teaspoons. His heart stopped beating around the time John got the spleen out; we shocked it, we paced it through the pacer cables, but Harvey got his wish. Ironically, had we left him alone, he might not have died, at least not right away. In over-riding his request, John gave him what he wanted.

Repairing abdominal aortic aneurysms has always been a big deal; more so back then because we (surgeons everywhere) were still working on the left side of the learning curve. The abdominal aorta supplies blood to everything below the diaphragm; screwing up the repair has serious consequences. Clamping off all flow below a certain point is required; how much depends on individual anatomy. If the clamp has to be placed above the renal arteries (to the kidneys), it doesn't take long for the kidneys to be damaged. Or grunge from within the aneurysm can get broken off in the process of repair and blast its way into the legs, or the intestines. (It's amazing and disgusting how much crud can pile up inside an aneurysm. Typically, it's a huge glob of meaty, yellowish, cheesy, gooey stuff, like something your dog vomited up, only firmer.) Worse, it can happen that a big thin aneurysm will blow during the operation, before full control has been achieved. Not good. So you'd be right if you imagined there was a certain amount of puckering going on within the sphincters of those involved in such operations.

Dr. Rockford admitted a patient with the biggest aneurysm anyone had ever seen. By definition, you can feel it on physical exam: a firm and pulsating mass in the mid-upper belly. But this was more: visible across the room, the top part disappeared up under the ribs. Clamping above the kidneys was inevitable, bursting was possible, a long operation with demanding post-op care unavoidable. And Rockford, undoubtedly, would be burning a short fuse. In fact, before the operation he tracked me down and said, ominously, "You better be scrubbed in on this case." Pucker went the ol' sphincter, enough to squeak.

Just as well. Otherwise, I'd have crapped in my pants.

When Rockford entered the OR, the patient was already prepped and draped, and the room was atypically populous: in addition to the usual retinue of residents, students, and the intern (me), word had gotten around, so a couple of research fellows and other surgeons were there to watch. Even the patient's own doc had come up from LA. Ignoring everyone in the room, Rockford walks in, gets gowned and gloved, bellies up to the table, asks for the knife. Looks me straight in the eye and . . . hands the knife to me. What was that?? I'd been on the service a few weeks, had made a scratch a couple of times in the OR, but never. . . . So there I was, in front of God and everyone, making a stem-to-stern incision, right over that enormous pulsating scary aneurysm. It was the most amazing thing that had happened to me so far (my part, of course, ended with the incision). And during the whole case, which went blissfully smoothly, it seemed Dr. Rockford spoke only to me, demonstrating technique, explaining his plan, as if I were his son and teaching me were his mission, his pleasure.

When it was over, I had to go to the surgery office. There sat an intern applicant, nervous and silent, enduring the delays and screwups that were par for the course for some reason in the UCSF interview process. I looked at him and sang out, "This is the greatest surgery program on the planet! I haven't slept in two days, but I just had the most exciting time in the OR imaginable. I love it! Good luck to you!"

There was another Rockford aneurysm case scheduled to follow the first, and I scrubbed back in, serenely awaiting the surgeon's arrival, ready to accept the next implied accolade. His eyes were black with animus from the moment he walked in, and he spewed at us all, berating me and everyone else for the whole two hours, for no reason I ever figured out. Heading back to the surgery office as soon as I was done, I found the poor supplicant still sitting there. "I take it all back," I said. "This place sucks, and if I were you I'd get the fuck out of here before it's too late."

At the end of the year, Ken Rockford had a party for the interns at his ranch. His cheerful and garrulous old dad was there, working and sharing a bulldozer which I drove all over the place, pulling the levers and pushing the brakes to make the thing spin on its tracks, a childhood fantasy fulfilled. When I was in Vietnam, Ken—alone among the professors—sent me a letter, and he included a picture of me, my soon-to-be wife, and his dad on the bulldozer.

I'll assume you aren't wondering how we took X-rays of people's aortas back then, but I'm going to tell you anyway, because it's a good story. There we were at UCSF Medical Center, at the leading edge (one of them, anyway) of vascular surgery; but instead of sending patients to the X-ray department for a semi-automated procedure—the radiologist threading a fine catheter up through a leg artery, mechanically taking films in rapid sequence like most everywhere else—we took them to the OR. Dr. Wylie insisted that the only way safely and accurately to image the aorta was to lay patients face down and poke a very long needle through their backs, angling in far enough away from the midline to skim past the spine and end up in the aorta. Inserting a needle to draw blood compares to that procedure the way a hook and string on a bamboo rod compares to fishing with dynamite: pushing a very large and long needle through those thick back muscles, hoping not to do an accidental kidney biopsy, feeling the needle start to bounce as it touches the aortic wall, confirming proper placement by observing a rhythmic squirt of blood across the room. Next to the patient's table, which was made of wood with a full-length slot under it, there would be another table stacked with six or eight X-ray plates which were nearly five feet long and a foot and a half wide. Then, as the end of the needle--sticking several inches out of the patient's back, and attached to a big syringe full of dye—flickered in time to the heartbeat, I'd stand between the two tables, bent and ready like a runner in starting blocks. After warning the patient to expect a hot sensation everywhere below the waist (Bugs Bunny in Elmer Fudd's boiling pot comes to mind), the resident would start pushing in the dye, and I'd shout to the X-ray tech (watching with amusement behind leaded glass), "SHOOT!" and begin a decidedly non-automated process of grabbing a plate, spinning around, shoving it under the patient, pushing the previous plate out the other side and into the hands of another human automaton, wheeling back for another, yelling "SHOOT" again, while God knows how much radiation sprayed the area. Spin grab spin push yell, spin grab spin push yell . . . getting as much film in and out as possible in about ten seconds. It felt like some sort of stupid game-show stunt, except that instead of winning a car, I got a set of testicles that glowed in the dark for two days. . . .

The Vascular Service is where I first got to know Jerry Goldstone. He was and is the nicest guy in all of academic surgery, anywhere, no question, hands-down, bar none, that's him. At the time, he was a fourth-year resident, smart, able, and supportive. "Schwab!" he'd say, "How the hell are you?" And he actually wanted to know. When there was more to do than I could get done, he'd pitch in, unlike anyone else at his level. He was there salving the wounds when we screwed up, giving perspective, taking our side. Of course, there was the little matter of his eyes. If I wondered what thyroid patients thought when they heard Lester Weisman's hoarse voice, it was unfathomable that people would allow Jerry to ream out the main blood supply to their brains. He'd look at you with one eye while the other gazed about thirty degrees out over your shoulder. And then it would be the other eye on you, while the first took flight. Whoa, could you find me another doctor, please? Assuming you can see him? I think it was because Jerry was so appealing, his empathetic smile and easy rapport making it clear that he would never do anything to harm anyone, that patients felt totally at ease and confident from the minute he met them. And it turned out that because he'd for his whole life alternated the use of each eye, he maintained equal acuity. Late in residency, he underwent surgery to straighten his eyes and defied the odds by gaining binocular vision. No idea why the hell he waited so long. Jerry and his wife Linda (a voluptuous beauty, ever with a laugh, among the world's best moms, an artist and activist) became and remain great friends. He's now Chief of Vascular Surgery at the University Hospital in Cleveland, where I went to med school. He's a superb teacher, leader, and researcher. How he stands the academic gamesmanship and backbiting, I will never understand.

seven

Heartstrings

The operator failed to call me at five a.m. as requested so I was a couple of minutes late for rounds to start my cardiac surgery rotation. I explained and apologized, embarrassed. "We begin on time around here," said Frank, the fourth-year, showing who's boss. Great start.

So far, I've bragged about how outstanding and prestigious were the departments through which I'd rotated. Manned by two strange surgeons, cardiac was the exception. David Williams was a paranoid lunatic. Chatham Knell was a patrician and elegant man who had made important contributions to open-heart surgery in his day, but no longer got very good results. Some called him Death Knell. It had become a sad cycle: as his practice ebbed, he still wanted to work, and he became willing to take on cases that no one else would have touched. High risk; hearts failing beyond salvage. No chance to live without surgery; maybe one in a hundred with it. Do such patients deserve a shot? I'll tell you this: no way they'd get it today. Data are published; mortality rates are in the public record. Surgeons need to cover their asses. The frail-hearted and the faint-hearted. Guess who loses. At least Knell gave them a chance.

Tall and slender, always well-dressed and wearing a fashionable thigh-length white coat, half-glasses studiously perched part-way down his nose, Dr. Knell had several teaching points he liked to make over and over. We heard the same things a million times, verbatim, as if he'd popped a tape into a slot in his head. That's what we called the speeches: cassettes.

Actually, that's what Joe Utley called them. Joe was the cardiac fellow—a fully trained general surgeon (he'd been in practice a few years before deciding to take up cardiac), now under the tutelage of those, uh, unique individuals. Incongruously for such a department, Joe was a superb surgeon and a wonderful guy. A Southern boy, Joe (full name: Joe) looked a little like Gomer Pyle, told corny jokes with a purse-lipped smile, played the flugelhorn. He'd seen the just-released movie *Patton* and liked to quote from the opening speech, which was something like "Many of you wonder if you'll know what to do in combat. When (here's the part Joe really liked and said with the proper

Try as I might, I can't rid my head of the vision of Joe wearing a sombrero, playing "Tijuana Taxi" the night he had me and Judy (future wife) over for dinner. In fact, I don't want to lose the image: Joe died recently, way too young. Like a friend in combat, I loved the guy.

gravity—I quote Joe exactly; whether it's cinematically accurate, I can't say) you put your hand in a glop of goo that used to be your best friend's face, you'll know what to do." Whenever there was a critically urgent admission, Joe would call me and say, for example, "Sid, we have a guy coming in with acute failure and an infected aortic valve. He'll need blood typed, an a-line, CVP, clotting studies . . . oh well, you'll know what to do."

We saw several of those emergency valve cases: heroin addicts had a way of squirting infected dope into their veins (often from a supply transported across the border in a balloon or condom in someone's rectum), and getting bugs growing on their heart valves.

For a while we had a study going to see if immediate replacement of the infected valve could salvage anyone from otherwise certain death. (Answer: nope. Sooner or later, they all got reinfected.) They were always a huge thrash: sick as hell pre- and post-op, they tended to bleed copiously in the OR, making an interminably long operation even longer, and were less than appreciative afterwards. Showing a poor prognostic sign, one young man tried to check out AMA (Against Medical Advice) from the ICU with his central line still in place, the new valve ticking his seconds away.

A central line is a long IV tube, placed either by cutdown or by piercing a jugular or other nearby vein, and threaded very close to the heart. Addicts, of course, had big problems finding their veins; a central line was like a gift from God.

I hated scrubbing on cardiac cases. With Chatham Knell in charge, they took forever, even if he was having Joe do the work. Each stitch was discussed, admired, evaluated before and after placing it. ("No, Joe, not there. That's it, that's good, ok, ok, yeah, right there, yeah, good. Good one, Joe. No, no, take it out. Do it again." X-rated stuff, if you listened with your eyes closed, as mine often were.) Thought and rethought excruciatingly, millimeter by millimeter, nothing was ok the first time. And this was after spending at least a couple of hours to get the patient on bypass (hooked up to the "heart-lung machine") and ready for the real operation. When it was Joe's case alone, as it was for clinic patients, things went more rapidly and well. Being a good surgeon has much less to do with flash and technical brilliance, than it does with being able to think ahead, be efficient, and know the shortest line between points A and B; in other words, having a certain type of decision-making capability. Much of it can be taught, I guess. But a critical portion is about how one's mind works. Like music. Some have it, some don't. Not everyone who lacks it chooses another profession.

It's surprising to note that in 1970, coronary bypass surgery—now by far the most common heart operation—was barely known. Nearly everything we did then was truly "open" heart: replacing valves, fixing holes between the chambers. Heart-lung machines, essential for such surgery, were likewise in the early stages of development, and quite damaging to blood cells. So the longer a patient was on bypass, the worse shape they'd be in after it was over: damaged blood doesn't clot, cell fragments clog up kidneys. Since being on bypass forever was a given with Knell's surgery, a rocky post-op course was typical, a fatality not rare. But it taught me a lot about managing all manner of heart problems. Once, when a patient developed a sudden rhythm problem in the middle of the night, I fixed it with no time to call for help and checked in with Joe afterward. As I explained to him what I'd done, I heard the sonorous sounds of sleep in the phone, as he drifted off. "Joe? Joe?" Quiet and slow, only breathing. So I hung up and went back to bed. About an hour later I got a STAT page from the operator: Joe had awakened with the phone in his hand and called in a panic wanting to know what the hell had happened. "Joe," I said, "I know what to do."

With the heart open and patient on the pump, the first time I scrubbed with Dr. Knell he asked, "Name seven reasons for oxygenated blood appearing in the left ventricle on bypass." Yikes! Not the sort of thing they cover in med school. This was a couple of days into the rotation, and I figured I'd be branded an idiot for the whole time. I spooled my mind through what little I could find: . . . uh, patent ductus? . . . let's see, uh . . . anomalous pulmonary venous return? . . . And then, behind Dr. Knell's head appeared a professionally plasticized cue-card, held up by the pump tech, with all the answers, readable across the room. Wow, I thought. This place is ok.

In addition to the pump techs, the team cardiologist John Hutchinson was always in the room. His presence was a bright spot in the otherwise dreary proceedings. He liked to talk, crack jokes, keep it light, especially if things were going awry. Hanging around surgeons agreed with him, and he admitted even his non-surgical patients to our care, believing that we, and the surgical nurses, paid more attention to them than did the internists and their crew. He was a pragmatist, a find-the-problem-and-fix-it sort of guy, which is not typical of medical types, who'd rather quote journals for an hour or two. Nowadays techs run the pump, but Hutch liked to do it himself; he looked so happy sitting at the controls, he should have been wearing goggles and a beanie. He transcended even that plane once, when we had a patient who wouldn't stop bleeding.

During bypass, blood thinners are given, and then reversed when the pump run is over. Sometimes, for many reasons, reversal isn't enough to achieve clotting. Blood products such as platelets and plasma are given, time passes, and usually it gets to the point that the chest can be closed. In one such instance, Joe actually scrubbed out and donated a pint of his own blood (his type matched the patient's): fresh blood has magic powers. In our case, nothing was working and it was starting to look like the patient might bleed forever. Without a goodbye, Hutch disappeared from the OR, to return a few minutes later wearing a feather headdress and carrying a rattle, which he held over the wound, chanting. Huyah, hiyah, huyah.... The bleeding stopped.

I believe I mentioned that Dr. Williams was a lunatic. He was a good operator but certifiably crazy in the OR, regularly losing control, yelling, berating people, throwing instruments. He might accuse someone of sabotage if something went wrong. That kind of crap was tolerated back then. Shaking his head like a bad imitation of Richard Nixon, he'd tighten his lips into a sort of cephalic anus and suck air in with a hiss at anything he didn't like, which was nearly everything. The ICU must have sounded like a steam room, as Joe and I walked around hissing at each other, imitating that simmering surgical sneer. David Williams was also the jealous type and couldn't stand the idea that anyone might be regarded more highly than he—especially not Joe, who clearly was.

Up from Louisiana, Orville Hatfield was a sweet old man who'd been on the ward for weeks while Williams tried to get him ready for an enormous operation. The poor guy couldn't eat and had a hole draining pus out of his chest. After poking him with scopes and exploring him with X-rays, Dr. Williams had concluded that Orville had an esophageal stricture (narrowing of the esophagus down to a thread) that had perforated, causing an infection which tracked through his lung and out to his skin. He'd need an esophageal replacement (remove the esophagus, and swing a section of intestine—usually colon—up into the chest, still attached to its blood supply in the belly, and then sew it as a conduit between neck and stomach) along with partial removal of a lung. Getting Orville, skinny and frail, through such a daunting operation would be nearly impossible, but he was pleasantly compliant and willing to undergo whatever it would take to get him back to dipping his feet in the Mississippi again. Sensing something amiss, Joe had reviewed all the charts and X-rays and drawn a very different conclusion: Orville had a Zenker's diverticulum— a pocket that develops in the upper esophagus, pooching outward toward the back of the neck. The esophagus itself is more or less normal, but food can head into the diverticulum, which then pushes against the esophagus, obstructing it. (One of Dr. Knell's cassettes involved a story about a man with a Zenker's who used to carry around a jar of pickled oysters. Before eating, he'd swallow one, which exactly filled the diverticulum without pushing too much on the esophagus. So he could eat, after which he'd push on the side of his neck and regurgitate the oyster into the jar. Probably didn't get invited out much.)

To confirm his diagnosis, Joe took Orville to the OR and again passed a scope down his throat. (Those were the days of rigid scopes; harder to maneuver and more error-prone than today's flexible fiber-optics.) He showed me: with excellent aim, you could get down a normal esophagus. Insert the scope less carefully—as Dr. Williams clearly had—and you were in the pouch, which dead-ended in such a way as to suggest a tight stricture. At its bottom was the tiny opening of the tract that led into Orville's chest and out to his skin—perforation being a known but infrequent complication of a Zenker's. Joe was practically dancing: he'd read of a procedure in which, if the diverticulum were lying right against the esophagus, you could make a couple of quick snips through the scope, eliminating the wall between them. No dead end, no stuck food. Two minutes, and Orville could head back to the Mississippi mud. But because of the way things worked, Joe couldn't just go ahead and do it, so he went to Dr. Williams, diplomatically to tell him what he'd found and how he proposed to fix it. Williams would not believe he'd been wrong, or that Joe's findings could be trusted. "You're not staff," was what he said, and he refused to schedule another procedure. YOU'RE NOT STAFF! What an arrogant prick! As he told me about it, Joe beat me on the shoulders with both fists. But he was undeterred. Staying with the radiologist while it was done, Joe got a live-motion X-ray, taking shot after shot until they finally got the dye to show what was going on. At our next weekly case-conference, Joe presented his findings, sweetly innocent, going over the head of a seething David Williams. Permission granted. Snip snip. Orville was chortling and chowing, free of drainage, toes twitching and ready to head south in about a week. Williams never forgave Joe.

One of the most catastrophic things that can happen in your chest is dissection of the aortic arch. Aiming first upward toward the head and then down to the belly, the aorta is shaped like a cane as it carries blood from the heart. The handle of the cane is the aortic arch, from which the main branches to the brain and the arms, as well as to the heart itself, head off before the aorta turns downward through the rest of the chest and to the abdomen. All blood vessels have layers which, under the wrong circumstances, can separate, allowing blood to worm its way between them. That's called "dissection." As it occurs, the layers further separate, pulling inward and away from the vessel wall, obstructing flow and plugging up branches along the way. It can happen anywhere along the aorta. When it happens in the arch, it may occlude flow to the brain or heart, in which case you likely won't make it to the phone. It can leak blood back into the sac (pericardium) around the heart, filling it up and compressing the heart (pericardial tamponade), usually splitting open the aortic heart valve in the process. If dissection is diagnosed before these things happen, it's possible to repair or replace the arch. But doing such a thing emergently and having a non-fatal outcome requires luck and skill and possibly divine intervention under the best of circumstances. The UCSF cardiac program was not, in my opinion, the best of circumstances in 1970–71.

The one arch dissection I saw came on the heels of a couple of monumental failures of the surgical approach, so we tried something else: studies had suggested that medically lowering the victims' blood pressure and keeping it that way for a couple of weeks or more allowed the aortic wall to resolidify, either avoiding surgery altogether or allowing a more controlled, non-emergency repair. When Carl Black came in with the typical searing chest pain boring into his back, and the aortagram confirmed the diagnosis, he was admitted to the ICU for controlled hypotensive therapy. Not as easy as it sounds: let the pressure get too low, and he'd stop making urine. Too high, and he'd have chest pain. Moreover, after a period of time the body can become resistant to various drugs, so it was a matter of dialing different doses of different drugs and dripping them in, walking a fine line day and night. The graphs looked perfect: between the other intern and me, we kept Mr. Black in the zone around the clock. We were rightly proud. And disappointed when he blew.

It was a day for the books—this book, as it turns out. A week or so earlier, a twelve-year-old girl had been admitted to the ICU, in respiratory failure from botulism. She wasn't on our service, but it was so unusual that we were well aware of her. Her initial treatment had been elsewhere, and included a tracheostomy. A low one. Out of metal.... We were making ICU rounds, Joe, Frank, and I, along with one of the attendings assigned to the ICU, Barry Singer, an anesthesiologist. Standing just outside the little girl's room, we noticed some movement and turned to see blood squirting from her neck, geysering nearly to the ceiling. We rushed into her room. While I stood replaying another similar scene, Barry and Joe acted with instinct for which there was no precedent: Barry somehow managed to pass a breathing tube through her mouth and into her trachea, despite the flood of blood pooling in his view. Joe yanked out her trach tube and inserted his finger into the hole in her neck, wiggling it down toward her chest along the front of her trachea, and when his finger found the innominate artery, he pushed it up against her sternum. The blood stopped. Amazing. It had never been done before; who knows how they came up with it. I helped wheel the bed to the OR, while Barry squeezed the Ambu bag (for assisting breathing) and Joe ran along with his finger in the tyke. Dr. Knell came to the OR to split the girl's sternum, expose the area, and fix it. A gloved finger looks a little like an artery, and Knell at first wasn't sure which he was seeing. Tapping on the structure didn't help: Joe's finger was by now numb as a post. Since compressing her artery hadn't caused a stroke, the solution was to tie it off. She did great, and in a few weeks recovered from her botulism, too.

They eventually published a report: it's the definitive way to control tracheo-innominate fistula. It works if the patient is in the ICU, with an anesthesiologist and cardiac surgeon standing within ten feet when it happens.

As the operation was ebbing, I got a STAT call to the ICU. I arrived in time to see Frank slashing open Mr. Black's chest. He'd crashed suddenly, losing all blood pressure. Because his neck veins were also markedly bulging, it meant he'd dissected back into his pericardium, causing tamponade. Frank made the call: open the chest, open the pericardium, and free the heart. But it wasn't going well. There was blood everywhere, dripping off the white curtains separating the beds, collecting along Mr. Black's side, pooling and ready to overflow the bed, while the monitor still showed no pressure. Bank blood arrived, and I started pouring it in. A crowd gathered: nursing students, med students, pharmacy students, agog, forming a half-circle of souls, like a Greek chorus, open-mouthed but silent. David Williams showed up, amok, shouting contradictory and useless orders while he was still in the hall. Then Joe arrived, fresh from saving the young girl, wanting the lowdown. "It looks like he dissected back into his pericardium and tamponaded," I told him. Williams wheeled around at me and snarled, "Of all the people in this room, you're the LEAST qualified to make that statement." Given my near round-the-clock attention to Mr. Black over the past days, that sort of pissed me off. Pointing to one of the pharmacy students, I said, "I think SHE'S less qualified, Dr. Williams." Joe elbowed me in the ribs, sharply. Carl Black died.

My first attempt on a patient's life came at three in the morning. I was called to the ICU to see a patient with pneumothorax (a collapsed lung), which had developed while on a ventilator—high pressures can sometimes pop a hole in a lung. The patient was a young kid with muscular dystrophy who managed independent breathing only until he got any sort of infection, even a cold. He was now in precarious shape, needing good care and better luck ever to breathe on his own again. I looked at the X-ray; there was a chest full of leaked air on the right. Frank, called in the wee hours, was happy to have me take care of it. Confidently, easily— having done this so many times in the ER—I inserted a tube in his chest to let the air out and re-expand the lung. Having ordered a followup chest X-ray, I told them to call me when it was done, and I headed back to bed. When the call came, the doc said, "You're not gonna believe this: now he has a pneumo on the other side."

Looking at the new pictures, it was obvious what I and everyone else had missed earlier: the original X-ray had been put up backwards. The kid's weakened muscles caused his back to curve, skewing his chest and displacing his heart to the right, and the air under pressure in the left chest had made the distortion even worse. Lots of people take a casual look at a chest X-ray and put it on the viewer making sure the heart is on the left, where it belongs; in this case, that casual move caused the X-ray to be flipped. Now, knowing which side the tube was on, it was apparent that the picture had been put up correctly. So there it was: the air pocket on the left, where it had been all the time. Horrified (and angry at the medical doc who'd made the original mistake, and at myself for missing it), I placed a second tube, believing I'd delivered a fatal blow—two of them—to the poor kid. With tubes on both sides, and possible damage to the lung from my original stab, he'd never get off the ventilator. When I told Joe of my error, I felt I'd let him down, undeserving of the faith he seemed to have in me. He just pointed out the obvious: always look at the Left/Right markers on the film. I always do, now. (And I've seen a couple of markers that were placed backwards.) The patient recovered, with difficulty, and went home again, breathing without assistance.

The rest of the days on cardiac were hardly as dramatic, but they were long and exhausting. I was a lone intern for a week when one of the other interns with whom I shared two-month rotations went on vacation. One afternoon, as I was napping in the little room at back of the ICU, Joe came in. I hadn't been home in days, and he evidently took some offense at my socks, which he managed to pull off and throw out the window before I was fully able to defend myself. I assumed it was an act of love.

Before moving on, I must say this about Chatham Knell: he was a tragic character, sometimes amazingly soulful. He'd talk to me, an intern of all things, about his frustrations as the cardiac world seemed to leave him behind. He took me out on his sailboat on San Francisco Bay one Sunday. I think life gave him a raw deal toward the end of his career. And one more thing—a few years later, when Dr. Dunphy retired, a new chairman was hired: Paul Ebert, a heart surgeon who specialized in children. There was quite a buzz around his arrival; he'd certainly turn the heart program around. The first case he did was an ASD repair (atrial septal defect: a hole between the upper chambers of the heart) in a child. I wandered into the OR to see the good part, having given him an hour and a half to get on bypass. He was closing.

"What, he couldn't do it?" I asked.

"No, he patched it up already," I was told.

"He did it without the pump?"

"No, we had a ten-minute run."

Wow. Things were never the same.

eight

A Bit of a Life

I'm sure I'd never have been an orthopedist, but sampling it right after cardiac sealed the no-deal. Cardiac surgery was (slashed chests to the contrary) delicate, thoughtful, quiet: carefully controlling the tiniest blood vessels before closing up. Meticulous and precise. Ortho was swinging sledgehammers, turning the cautery unit up to well-done, charring tissues like the Fourth of July. Cringed into the back of my mind, my memories of the month are few. To wit: total hip replacement was just appearing. The fancy brackets and braces now used to hold the devices were nonexistent, so we interns had to sling the leg over our shoulders, lean back, and pull through the whole damn operation. An even more unpleasant recollection is being asked to get an op-permit from an unfortunate and bitter man whose previously placed rods in his spine had broken and needed replacing. Worse, during the first operation, he'd been given the wrong type blood and nearly died. Knowing zilch about rodding backs, I walked into the room to get the permit, at which point he placed a tape recorder in front of me and punched "start." I moon-walked back out and called the resident. Oh, and I got pretty good with orthopedic plaster. I stole a few rolls, and Judy (she's coming right up) and I used them to make a life-size figure of an old man wearing a vest. We bought a pocket watch, put it in the vest-pocket, added a pair of glasses, and gave it to some friends as a grandfather clock.

The passing by of ortho, wasted, seems a good time to mention that I managed to have part of a life outside the hospital. San Francisco, 1970. Went to a movie right after I arrived, *Mad Dogs and Englishmen* (best concert movie ever, with Joe Cocker and Leon Russell), and people were tapping me on each side, passing joints up and down the aisle. How bad could this be? The Summer of Love was a faded tie-dye memory, but Haight-Ashbury was right around the corner from UCSF. One weekend I volunteered at the Haight-Ashbury Clinic—an icon in '60s lore, the quintessential free clinic which cared for thousands of kids and set a standard for the rest of the country. Maybe I thought it would prove me cooler than the typical surgeon. If I met a free-loving hippie, that would be ok, too. It didn't occur to me until I checked in that any flower children still in the Haight in 1970 were too burnt-out to have noticed that everyone else had left. Expecting some sort of professional and/or personal satisfaction, instead I saw a couple of cases of gonorrhea in too-young and too-sad girls, and a circumferential blister from a flea-collar belt, fashioned by a young lady sleeping somewhere on a bare mattress. Clearly, I was way too late. Not needing voluntary sadness, I didn't go back.

Two friends from college, Rick and Tim, were living in San Francisco. When I could stay awake, I spent some time with them. (My brother Doug and his wife Lis lived there, too. That's how busy I was: I hardly ever saw them.) Shortly after I arrived in San Franciso, Rick said, "Hey Schwab, guess who's moving here?"

"Who?" I asked, too tired for games.

"Mumma!" [Pronounced "MOO-muh"]

"...?..."

"You know, from the party in Cambridge." Oh, yeah—Rick had talked me into driving from Cleveland to Cambridge one weekend for a party (he'd gone to Harvard law school after Amherst), and to meet a girl, Judy Mumma, a Harvard undergrad. We'd had a nice time, no fireworks. She seemed more interested in Rick than in me. I filed the fact of Judy's impending arrival and didn't think much more about it.

In medical school, after breaking up with a fellow student with whom I'd had a much too complex relationship, I met Diane, who wanted a no-strings, see-me-when-you-have-time sort of thing. Perfect. We stayed in touch, and she came to visit me in San Francisco. Suddenly she wanted more strings than the suture chairs. Anxious for diversion, I took her to a gathering that Rick was having at his family place in Dutch Flat, up in the Sierras: a rustic white-painted, big-porched home dating back to the Gold Rush. Diane and I went for the weekend, having a lousy time, aware of but ignoring the inevitable. The party was well under way when we arrived, so we walked through Rick's empty house and out into the back yard, into a group of mostly familiar people. And there was Judy Mumma, swimming in a pond with her black lab Jake. We laughed as Jake pawed at her while Judy hollered and splashed. Drowning, as it turned out. Rick's cousin recognized that the cries were not from joy, swam out and pulled her in. I helped her ashore. Hi, I'm Sid. Remember me? Howya doin'? Want some CPR? The connection that Cambridge had lacked seemed to happen in Gold Country.

Judy is the most unscrewed-up person I've ever met. She was working on a master's degree in education from Claremont and had come to San Francisco to be a student teacher. She's smart and artistic, an omnivorous lover of life. Unselfish and comfortable with herself, she's the friend you wish you had. She cut up colored cellophane and turned the windows in my apartment door into stained glass. When I was stuck in the hospital, she'd bring food over and we'd picnic in a call room. When there was time, we found great hole-in-the-wall restaurants, went to shows, made the most of it; and she had a million things she did when I wasn't around. Happy with his matchmaking, Rick celebrated with an ad in the personals of the *San Francisco Chronicle:* "Schwab, all is forgiven. Please return dentures. Mumma." Herb Caen, whose column in the *Chronicle* was legendary for decades, picked up on it and wondered in print what it all meant. "I admire terse writing, but this cries for an explanation," he wrote. Rick contacted Herb Caen and gave him my number along with some personal info about me and Judy. Trying to be truthful, I explained to the assistant who called me (by paging me through the hospital operator—theretofore reserved for emergencies) that it was a joke, just the latest of the many "bits" Rick liked to pull, intended only to get a laugh, having to do with nothing; but that's not what he wanted to hear. So I concocted wooden dentures, an heirloom, grabbed after an argument. A couple of days later, Mr. Caen wrote in his column, something like: "Remember that personals ad? Our sleuths have solved the mystery. Turns out Schwab is a 6'4" ex rugby player from Amherst, now a surgery intern at UCSF. Mumma is 4'10", out of Harvard, former mascot for the Boston Patriots, now a teacher. Schwab ran off with the dentures, a family heirloom, after a lovers' spat. Once again the *Chronicle*

Cutting Remarks

True, mostly. While at Harvard, Judy was hired by the team to wear a Paul Revere outfit and run around the stands cheering for the Pats. But she's darn near five feet tall. I got a call from a lab doc at the hospital wondering if the Caen column was accurate. I said not the part about the dentures. He meant her height. He had a daughter in the Little People of America, and they'd love to hear from a little person who'd made good. Thanks again, Rick.

ads work; they're back together." Next day, I passed Dr. Wylie in a hospital hallway. "Goddamn sex maniac," he growled. "You need to work harder."

nine

Treating Veterans, and Becoming One

The most gorgeous real estate on the planet is occupied by the Veterans' Administration Hospital in San Francisco, its complex of buildings sparing a few nearly pristine acres at the very northwest corner of the peninsula. You can climb over a ledge and view the land as it has been for eons, untouched. West over the Pacific, toward the Farallone Islands; north across the Golden Gate to the barren and brown rolling Marin Headlands—you'll see wind-carved scrubby trees and rocky cliffs, hear the churning gray surf, sometimes the bark of sea lions, absent the hand of man, for miles and miles. A window in the respiratory ICU captured much of that vista, along with a view of the Golden Gate Bridge. Below the sill were rows of vets in bed, nicotine-scorched lungs huffed by ventilators, unaware of their good fortune. I'll go there when it's my turn. It was a struggle to pay attention on rounds.

The Chief of Surgery at the VA, Larry Way, trained at UCSF, so he had the expected amount of demanding uptightness. But really, you can't rush the VA; no matter how much surgical straining at the system, it moves at its own speed. Get an X-ray after 4 p.m.? Forget it. Order a potassium level? What do you mean,

Cutting Remarks

doc? You got one of those yesterday. Emergency surgery? Practically no such thing. Patients came there expecting to camp out for the winter at least, so there was no hurry to get them shaped up. Plenty of time to enjoy the view, likely to get home at night. A gentlemanly rotation. Larry cracked the whip, but it lacked a certain snap.

It was consensual. We'd give the men a place to stay, three decent meals, dry them out from their alcoholism when they'd run out of money; in return, they'd offer up their bodies for our pleasure. This was one place that I got to do a bit of surgery. I fixed a few hernias, got to do little parts of some bigger operations such as dissect along the outer edge of the colon, clamp cut and tie a vessel or two. Dr. Way had a thing about doing all hernias under local, and having the patient get off the table and walk to the recovery room. Showy. First time I tried it, I'd managed to let some local anesthetic leech its way around a major nerve to the leg, so the man couldn't stabilize his knee for a couple of hours. Flopped around for a few seconds before we put him back on a gurney. Embarrassing. I didn't even know that could happen.

Pete Phillips had taken a shotgun, aimed it at his heart, and pulled the trigger with his toe. Missing his chest, he blew away his spleen, part of his colon, stomach and pancreas, and his left kidney. That was a few years earlier. Several operations

I mean no disrespect for veterans. I'm one myself. But there was, at least at that time, a fairly large group of vets who depended on the VA Hospital for more than simple medical care. They were down on their luck, broke, many of them alcohol- and nicotine-addicted. They really did make the rounds of VA hospitals in the country, moving with the weather; and in contrast to today, when funding and care are being drastically reduced, no one thought twice about parking a veteran in a room for a few weeks, drying him out, fattening him up, getting him ready for an operation if he needed one, or just helping him out if he didn't.

later he'd recovered but was left with an enormous hernia of his upper left abdominal wall, sticking out like an off-center backpack, containing much of his remaining innards. I'd seen him in the out-patient clinic and presented him to the attending surgeon, who agreed that the man was in no shape to undergo surgery; he was malnourished and drunk, among other things. Pretty much anywhere else, Pete would have been out of luck, but being the VA, we admitted him, fed him, dried him out. He tuned up just before I was finished with the rotation, and we managed to schedule his operation in the nick of time. The attending was a surgeon from Marin County who gave a lot of time helping at the VA. Not of the full-time UCSF mold, he was willing to let me do the case.

Abdominal wall hernias run the gamut: little holes here or there requiring a couple of stitches, mostly through predictable anatomic holes; or bulges through defects in a previous incision; or weird things, as in this case, requiring a certain make-it-up-as-you-get-there approach. By definition, a hernia means there's a hole somewhere with something pushing through it. What's pushing through, how stuck it is, how complex a repair is required can vary greatly. It might easily be an "intern's case," or it could test the skills of the most tenured professor. This one was pretty tough. Over my head, largely. But to the extent that I was given a chance to dissect things and put them back together again, even with a great deal of help, it was just what I needed. Finally a chance to see what I could do, and how I liked it. Rather than feel inadequate, which I was, I saw that

Surgeons who might read this are laughing with incredulity. It's impossible, they must think, that a training program would allow its interns to do so little, even more unbelievable that the interns would get so excited over a hernia. I agree. But there it is.

I'd actually learned a whisper of technique, had the ability to hold instruments without dropping them, and found the challenge exciting rather than daunting. It was a sign that I was on the right track. I liked this stuff, and I thought there was a chance I'd actually be able to do it someday.

The urology resident tried to sell me on the specialty, saying it could serve a surgeon perfectly for his whole career. When you were young and willing, he said, you could do big operations—total removal of the bladder, for example, with creation of a new one from intestine. The Bricker procedure. We did a few that month: big, indeed. When you wanted to slow down, you could do more predictable and less demanding things, like removing a kidney, or even less: carving out a prostate. Did some of that, too. And when you were too tired to do much of anything, you could have a useful office practice. As opposed to the general surgeon, for whom it is much more of an all-or-nothing deal. Made sense. Not ready to commit. On the service, I learned how to do vasectomies, which was fun. On the other hand, there was a patient, around twenty, who kept coming in having stuffed things up his penis and into his bladder. Thermometers, straws, pens and pencils. Crayons. Really annoying.

But most of all, there was the matter of the letter from Sam.

I came home one evening and checked the mail. Greetings from my government. Of all the interns in the UCSF programs—including medicine, surgery, and several others, there were around a hundred—only two of us got drafted. Mainly because I had just been accepted as a resident, it wasn't good news. I'd applied for the Berry Plan (a deferment of residents until fully trained, in exchange for an obligation to serve) but was told they were full. Since many of the older residents had gotten into the

Berry Plan, I'd asked Dr. Dunphy what he thought I should do. In the search for an exit strategy, the Vietnam War was in transition: Nixon was trying to "Vietnamize" it, reducing the number of Americans stationed there. Dunphy had been pretty sure the doctor draft was coming to an end, and because he was rumored to have connections in the Pentagon, I'd stopped worrying. Pleading hardship because they couldn't get new residents at this late date, the hospital wrote letters to each of our draft boards. The other intern's board wrote back and said, sorry, didn't mean any trouble, we take it back. Mine said, who are you kidding? At that point, upset as I was about losing my residency slot, I resigned myself to going; were I able to wriggle out, someone else would have to go in my place. But I wasn't happy. (Dunphy wasn't all that upset. He said, "War is good for surgeons." He also said they'd hold a place for me.)

The night I got the letter, we went bowling with friends—who wouldn't, after life rolls you a gutter ball? It was a miserable evening. Shell-shocked, I was bad company, while my friends forced lightness, avoiding the subject. How 'bout that Willie McCovey? Judy's usual positivity was absent.

Joe Utley told me I should get into the Air Force and become a flight surgeon. It was fun, he said, and flying status paid more. He had the name of an officer at the Presidio—the big Army complex in San Francisco. Trusting Joe with my life, I called the man and asked to be an Air Force Flight Surgeon, and that's what happened. Another ex-Air Force resident told me to call a Colonel at Lackland AFB in San Antonio, saying he's in charge of medical assignments. I did, and he was. "Would you like to go to Vietnam?" the Colonel asked.

"What else you got?" I replied.

"Want to go to the Philippines?"

"Well, actually, I'm getting married." (I hadn't really brought it up, but figured I would someday—technically not a lie.) "Plus there's this residency thing. I'd like to stay in the States. How about Hamilton?" (Hamilton AFB was in Marin County; I could go to conferences, keep my face known at UCSF.)

"OK," he said. "Call me in three days, and I'll let you know."

Wow, what a great guy. I basically told him I didn't want to go to Vietnam, and he didn't make me feel like a slacker. Phu Kat, Vietnam, is where he assigned me.

There were 130 in my group in Flight Surgeon School, including many single guys, of whom several had said they *wanted* to go overseas. I was the only one assigned to Vietnam, the only one leaving the U.S.

I wasn't to report to Brooks AFB in Texas for flight surgeon training until September. Judy and I had been getting along pretty well; we had raised the possibility of marriage. Clearly I'd never find anyone as perfect as she, but it was a little soon for a commitment. On the other hand, going away for a year might let her slip away. Did it make sense to get married and head off to war? Who knows. We went for it. It's not as if I hadn't made all my other major life decisions without a clue of what I was doing. (Thirty-four years of marriage, it's been, and counting.)

We drove up to Portland, where my folks lived, and then to Bellingham, Washington, to see her family. When my parents met Judy in San Francisco, it had gone well. Everyone liked everyone. This was my first view of Judy's family—a large one, her mom and dad having produced eight girls and a boy. Most were still at home, in a twenty-room, turn-of-the-(last)-century house overlooking Bellingham Bay. Originally the home of a lumber baron and mayor, the place more recently had been a retreat for an order of nuns, who'd customized it for a houseful of females. Prior to that, the Mummas had been in various shacks, the projects, sometimes three to a bed, while her dad went to med school (selling brushes door-to-door to make money) and later learned to be an anesthesiologist. Now there was a bedroom for each kid, multiple stalls and sinks in the bathrooms. They were in heaven, even without the nuns. When we told her parents we'd decided to get married, her dad slapped Judy on the back and said, "Way to go!" I took that as an ok.

We married in the ballroom of the Mumma house, Judy wearing a muslin dress and I a fluffy shirt she'd made. As we walked in, my friend Dougie played "Here Comes the Sun" on the guitar; the song still moves me. Next day, we made for San Antonio in our new red 1971 BMW 1600, for which I'd traded my beloved but disintegrating Mustang. Everything we owned, except for books, was with us in that car. Arriving tired in San Antonio, we hurried our way into a crummy little corner of a four-plex, and I set about learning what a doctor needs to know about caring for fliers. What I remember most is how much the gas in your colon expands when you go up in an altitude chamber, wondering what it would be like to walk by when they vented the thing. And that doctors are pussies: we had to do such things as be gassed (tear gas, with and without masks) and give ourselves injections of fake antidote. About

The salesman from whom I bought the car was a Nazi. When I gave him my name, he asked me if I was Jewish. I was incredulous. More so when he said, "I'm not rezponzible for vat happened over dere." If I hadn't liked the car so much, I'd have taken the moral high ground and walked out.

half the guys could not make themselves jam a needle through their pants into their thighs (what, no alcohol swab??). Being the only one headed to war, I had no problem. All the stuff we did was fun—ejection seat and parachute trainers, water-survival. Kids playing grownup. They made us march. The drill-leader finally threw down his hat and walked off the field. Bunch a' doc draftees, figuring what are they gonna do, fire us?

Expecting to hate it—because that's what our friends who'd been there had done—Judy and I liked San Antonio. We found cool little restaurants along the river, camped on Padre Island, checked out Austin, and were mesmerized by spectacular storms of cloud lightning which illuminated dark stones in a cobbled sky, one at a time, now here, now there, as soft rumbles bounced over our heads, sounding impossibly far away. After three months, we reloaded the car and headed west, stopping for a ten-second look at the Grand Canyon, getting more and more silent as we neared Travis Air Force Base, gateway to Southeast Asia.

It started to get serious in the Philippines. Everyone on flying

---

We spent a night in the jungle, learning survival techniques. Broken into small groups, we had an Air Force leader, and a Negrito guide. The Negritos are a pygmy race, whose brilliant and ferocious assistance of the Marines trying to get the Japanese off the islands during WWII is legendary. Our guide knew everything: how to get water from a palm tree, which sap to use to stop bleeding, how to cook taro in a section of bamboo. In less than two minutes he made fire, starting with nothing but another piece of bamboo and a pocket knife: two surgical slices to fashion a bow, another to make a rod to spin with the bow, then several curls of bamboo flakes peeled up but still attached to the wood, in the middle of which to work the rod. A couple of puffs from his cheeks, and then there was fire. Our GI leader told us we could hide in hollows in the jungle floor. Someone asked about snakes. "There are no snakes," he said. "The Negritos think there are, but there aren't." Right. This man who just made fire out of nothing, who carries in his genes the status in the Air Force who was headed to Vietnam stopped there for jungle survival school. Escape and evasion. Edible plants. Torture resistance. Guy asked me where I was headed. Danang. Oh, he said. Rocket City.

I was still in my starchy khakis with my shiny silver captain's bars on the flight from Saigon to Danang. Sitting in a sling along the wall of a C-130 filled with Marines in full battle gear, smiling a don't-hurt-me smile, I probably looked like lunch.

When I arrived at Danang Airbase, I was greeted by the hospital administrator, a big gap-toothed major, surrounded by red hair. He gave me a ride from the airstrip to the clinic in a jeep, past guard towers, rolls of concertina wire, F-4 fighter-bombers screaming overhead, choppers throbbing on the horizon, over jungle trying to green its way back onto the asphalt. I don't recall having much to say, just looking around, shaking my head, already counting the days. The major and I got along ok, but he cracked and went home a few months later. Whereas the other docs lived in a hootch in the center of the base, with nurses next door, I

---

knowledge of a thousand generations in the jungle: ignore, we were told, his fear of the hollows. Needless to say, I stayed out of them. That was but one of several experiences with Asian cultures which confirmed that we in the West have much to learn. On the mother of all picnics, in a grotto above a monastery in central Thailand (as the North Vietnamese marched into the South at the ending of the war, we had to bug out of Danang, and spent the last couple of months in Thailand), I watched a young and never-schooled Thai woman climb a tree and shake it, calling the wild monkeys, who arrived tenatively, warily taking the pineapple chunks we tossed their way. "You be here before, do this?" I asked. "No, be here today, first time." "How you know call monkey?" "I know they come. I think, before, man, monkey be same-same." "You mean man live same like monkey?" "No. Man, monkey, same-same." Think what Darwin might have accomplished, had he been born Thai, in the jungle.

lived with the pilots, next to the flight line. Gunfighter Village, it was called. Prime target. My home was a two-story barracks, with concrete bunker walls around it, extending only to just below the top floor. Which is where my room was. I became able to sleep through the takeoffs and landings of fighter jets, but never the whoomp of rockets, landing somewhere far away and walking their way in, one after another. After a direct hit, I slept under the bed for the rest of my war.

So here's a few random memories from Vietnam. 1) Air Force pilots are phenomenal guys. I'd trust them to fly me anywhere in anything. 2) The war made no sense whether you were for it or against it. We got rocketed every day or night; each morning we'd be told how many rockets were being set up to fire at us. Couldn't do anything about them because they were in "friendly villages," which meant our troops needed permission from the village chief to enter. Had he granted permission, the chief would be dead by morning. 3) I learned more than I ever wanted to know about venereal diseases I'd never even heard of. (Guy tells me, hey doc, you treated me for the clap last week and it's back. I ask, what do you have, the burning or the drip? The drip, he says, taking down his pants to reveal his underwear with a green wet circle on the front, the size of a salad plate. Wow, that's a hell of a drip, I say. Yeah, he says. And that's just since Thursday. It was Tuesday.) 4) China Beach is spectacularly beautiful. I got there a couple of times, until the ride over (in an ambulance) became too dangerous. While we swam, helicopters patrolled above the shoreline, gunners dangling their feet out the open doors as they manned machine guns. 4a) Watching a nurse peeling off camouflage fatigues down to a bikini is among the sexiest things on Earth. 5) When the ARVN (the South Vietnamese soldiers) were in charge of base security, it was like a sieve. When the Marines or ROKs (South Korean—Republic of Korea—soldiers, the scariest guys in Southeast Asia) were around, things got real quiet. 6) I got hurt when that rocket hit my barracks, right before going on leave to Hong Kong to meet Judy. I managed ok with one arm in a sling. Because I'd cared for several injured before addressing my own wounds, the medics put me in for a Purple Heart, with which the hospital commander surprised me at a squadron meeting weeks later. Being in charge of medevac flights out of our base, I'd seen plenty of guys more severely injured than me, which made the award a little embarrassing. However, I have a Purple Heart license plate now, figuring if I get stopped for speeding, it couldn't hurt. 7) One of the docs taught me a better way to do vasectomies than I'd learned at UCSF, which was the first clue that maybe there's more than one right way to do a thing. I did tons of vasectomies in Danang, which seems strange. 8) I got to fly a lot of planes, and got fairly good at take-offs and landings. My roommate for a while was the chief instructor pilot for a squadron of EC-47s; I went along for some checkout rides, and he taught me a thing or two. I planned to get certified when I was back in the U.S. for my second year, but decided against it after being in a crash which totaled the little Cessna—flipped over and dripping gas from the wing-tanks—flown by a former helicopter pilot, now a real-estate salesman trying to sell me something. I figured I'd have less time than he to keep current. 9) On the day Nixon announced that the last Marines were out of Vietnam, Danang was still crawling with them. But they were officially stationed in the Philippines, in 'Nam on "temporary duty." That's how things worked. 10) Living closest to the hospital, when the rockets would drop in at night, I'd put on a flak jacket and helmet and run down the street to get there first, while Cobra helicopters strafed the surrounds of the base, tracers lighting up the jungle. Crazy. 11) I had it way better than most of the guys who served in Vietnam.

My second year in the Air Force was spent at McChord AFB, in Tacoma. We had more docs than we needed, and a hospital commander who mainly wanted to be with his girlfriend (his wife was in Texas) and who said we could run the show however we wanted as long as he didn't hear complaints. Judy and I found a tiny shack, one house back from the shore of Lake Steilacoom, a serene treasure still a few years removed from overdevelopment. It had a bedroom so small we had to get in and out of the same side of the bed. We loved it. I took lots of time off—if someone came to visit, I called and said I wouldn't be in, and people would cover. Having done time in Vietnam, I didn't feel guilty; none of the other docs had. We walked around the lake, hung out on a bridge where old men fished, took a carpentry class in which we made a cutting board and a table. It was a time in between breaths. For once free of consuming work, or of looming war, we were together as we'd not yet been.

part

The Middle

two

ten

Good as Gold

After nine months of idyll, my side of our little Beemer pulsated with silent tension, in time with the clenching of my jaw, as we drove over the Bay Bridge into San Francisco. From quiet walks around a lake to blaring horns, overloaded traffic, and the prospect of endless work, I felt the pressure squeeze the minute we made landfall. A couple of weeks later it occurred to me that I no longer noticed; one resets the dial to a different level of normal. No wonder we die young.

During internship, Jerry and Linda Goldstone had introduced us to Dan and Del, a gay couple next door who'd been together for years (and remained so until Del died, many years later). They were three-piece-suit guys, realtors, who owned apartments and lived in a neat little house on Cole Street, up the hill from the med center. Because they needed the rent to renovate their apartments, the house would be ours. (Two years later we bought it.) It was one of those wooden frame homes built right after the 1906 earthquake. Tidy and solid, a one-story, nine-hundred-square-foot "charmer" on a twenty-five-foot-wide lot, it had a garish and altogether lovable gilded mirror covering an entire wall of the living room, and an unexpectedly private and lavish back yard, over a hundred feet deep, terraced, with a huge cypress tree and a pond. The yard abutted a barren shoulder of Tank Hill, which looked like Arizona and conferred a feeling of solitude and peace. To step out the back of the house onto the little deck was to have traversed space and time. Safe, silent, and sunny. Many times the San Francisco fog stopped at our front door, magically leaving our garden to us. The house wasn't ready the day we arrived; Dan and Del put us up in one of their apartments. We found a bottle of wine in the fridge, a rose and a candle on the dining room table. Did you ever have landlords like that? Our house on Cole Street was a perfect place from which to relaunch training, but I worried that in two years, I'd forgotten everything I knew and lost the ability to work so hard. I hadn't.

✶

Being a first-year resident is like being an intern, but with fewer excuses. You're close enough to the bottom rung that from a distance it looks like you're still on the ground. You dip from the same pool of work to be done, but on some occasions you get away with telling an intern what to do. And you're a little more likely to get chewed out if something is overlooked. On the other hand, you get to do a bit more in the operating room.

I started on the Gold Service, which was the staff service at UC Hospital. The patients didn't have private doctors but were in the UC Clinic system, dredged up by us as we manned the out-patient surgery clinic. See a patient, evaluate the presenting problems, check it out with a senior resident or attending, and, if a surgical problem were diagnosed, admit the patient for a planned operation. We all split time between the in-patient wards and the out-patient clinics. The chief resident was in charge of figuring out who was assigned where at what time, and which patients would be admitted, had his pick of which he'd operate on, and which he'd pass on to less senior residents. During the time an attending was assigned to the Gold Service, he admitted his private patients there; otherwise Gold was one of only two services in the UC system in which the operations were generally nonemergent and were the charge of the resident staff.

One of my first patients was a large diabetic woman who'd gotten a massive infection of her belly wall from giving herself a careless insulin injection. She'd already had the infected tissues cut away, leaving her with an actual-size square foot of absent skin and fat, bottoming out at the muscle layer. Over the next two months I witnessed the power of the body to heal itself: the formation of "granulation tissue" (the "proud flesh" of olden days—the beefy red and healthy healing tissue that forms in wounds). Once there's a clean base of granulation, you'd have to try hard to get it infected; and it slowly contracts, bringing the wound edges together. She'd had a couple of failed attempts at skin grafts—they kept floating away in a sea of surface pus—so the process was allowed to carry on unaided. And eventually the entire crater was gone, smoothed over with a nice layer of skin. It made me realize that in no way are doctors healers: at our best, we optimize conditions, tilt the balance in the body's favor, so it can heal itself.

No contradiction: surface contamination isn't an infection, in the sense of danger to the patient.

Manning the clinic was—like so much else—mixed. We saw it as checking the traps: what could we find to haul into the hospital and operate on? Those people that came in for operations had to have their problems sorted out, explained, choices of therapies made. Not unlike the days of taking calls from my patient family in medical school, clinic involved creative stalling while I talked things over with a more senior resident or the attending. And learning that "textbook cases" were just that: how a disease was described in a book was unlikely to be the way it showed up when you stuck it in a human being and shook it around for a while. As interns, we had spoken derisively of the "LMD"—the Local M.D.—who'd so misdiagnosed and screwed up the case we'd admitted for proper care at the Medical Center, the Temple of Truth. Now (and before this, during my two years as a primary care doc in the Air Force) I began to realize that most belly aches are just belly aches. Flu-like symptoms are usually due to the flu. It's harder than I thought to separate out the more serious things; and you can't order a bunch of tests on everyone who walks through the door with a few hours of nausea. Rare things are rare; common things are common.

In clinic, I learned an important lesson: keep your eye on the audience. Following up on a prior operation, a man came in for suture removal, accompanied by his partner. Both insisted the partner be there to hold the patient's hand. Bending to the task, taking out the first stitch, I caught sight of movement but reached out too late for a save as the partner keeled over, straight as a felled tree, head arcing in a perfect quarter-circle, bouncing once, and settling on the concrete floor. He was discharged a few days later with only a concussion, and with a nice row of sutures in the back of his head which I'd placed—and later removed in the clinic—while his friend waited in the lobby.

Without a tray of sterile crochet-hooks, clinic would not have functioned. Forget about diagnosis of disease: our real role was to fish out infected sutures. At a teaching hospital, most big operations had at least two more people scrubbed in than was necessary, and the operations took hours too long. Bugs had lots of hosts from which to jump into the wound, and lots of time to do it. Bodies are able to rid themselves of minor infections, but not when there's foreign material in the middle of it. Plus, the suture material used for deep closure in those days was likely to generate a reaction, even absent infection. Coarse silk threads, even cotton; Dacron, too. Absorbable sutures at that time were generally too flimsy and transient to be used to hold abdominal muscles together. So we saw belly after belly lined with red protrusions like teats on a mommy pig, draining or ready to drain pus. Happily, you could root around at the bottom of the hole without causing much pain; the reaction probably gobbled up some nerve endings in the process. Insert the crochet-hook, twist and pull and scrape, pull back (sometimes with disturbing force), and out comes a stinky stitch. Well, I thought, this certainly sucks. Spend a few years as a surgeon, have a line of patients out the door and around the block, producing new sores faster than you could empty out the old ones. No time to do anything else.

Of course, a surgeon finishing training today wouldn't recognize a crochet hook if you stuck it up his nose: we now have strong-as-steel dissolving suture that lasts a few months, more than long enough for everything to heal, and then is gone. Wounds spitting out suture are history. Funny thing is, like many other surgical truths inculcated at the end of a whip during training, switching to using those materials caused a nearly-physical sense of wrongdoing. You can't spend several years hearing Dr. Dunphy tell you over and over why every wound ought to be closed with 2-0 silk without a pang of guilt as you abandon it for something that makes a hell of a lot more sense. Suture material is the least of it. There's very little I do now that's as it was during training, whether it be materials used, techniques, or post-op management. In the last several years, concepts that had flowered for decades have been uprooted and tossed out like weeds.

At some point, between plucking sutures from wounds and cleaning remnants of patients' friends off the floor, I managed to find my very own gallbladder patient and convince her that it was safe to be admitted and have me operate.

Your liver does dozens of manufacturing jobs; among its products is bile—a yellow liquid that helps you digest fat. About a quart per day is produced in the liver and drips steadily into your intestine through a tube called the bile duct. A small amount—a few tablespoons—is diverted into a storage pouch called the gallbladder, a little bag which hangs from under the liver. When you eat fat, the gallbladder squeezes an extra dose of bile into the gut. It's a nice plan, probably more important in the time when humans went days between kills: during starvation the gallbladder can get huge. If you eat half a buffalo, enough to last til the next time you find one, it's nice to have stored a blast of bile. But since we eat regularly nowadays, several times a day, constantly dripping bile works perfectly well. The good news for gallbladder patients and their surgeons is that in the vast majority of cases, storing bile isn't necessary and people get along just fine without their gallbladders. The bad news is that bile is a complicated liquid, which can form crystals in certain situations as it sits in the gallbladder. The crystals grow like sugar candy on a string, forming stones, which can cause an impressive list of problems: most commonly, intermittent severe pain; sometimes jaundice (turning yellow from bile backing up into the bloodstream) or infections. My patient had had several episodes of pain and was more than happy to separate herself from her gallbladder. Fixing hernias is surgery, but it's right there under the skin. Taking out an appendix is working in the belly, which is where the action is for a general surgeon, but it's a small thing. A gallbladder, well, that's stepping into the big time, at least for a first-year resident at UCSF. Even more so in those days of open surgery and monster incisions.

Unless it's not. Many is the family doc who took out an appendix or two in residency, only to find out later, on his own, how hard it can be under some circumstances. Appendectomy is your basic interns' case, in which you learn a bit about handling bowel, putting stitches in the colon (to which the appendix is attached), in a situation not usually very threatening. But it's also a laboratory for judgment, and if the appendix is very inflamed, or ruptured, or stuck behind the colon, it can be a major challenge to handle properly. No intern would ever be doing an appy without a very senior resident or attending at hand.

The top of the gallbladder is close to the undersurface of the abdominal wall, but the rest of it lives down deep, with the attachments that need dividing hunkering close to the backside, near some serious anatomy: the main arteries and veins to the liver, the bile duct, the pancreas. Depending on how inflamed the gallbladder is or has been, identifying and protecting those structures can be a piece of cake, or a cold-sweat-inducing nightmare. It helps to know how to handle tissues, both normal and abnormal, how to dissect, how to avoid trouble. Not to mention cutting and tying in a deep hole. I knew little about those things, but you have to start somewhere, and having an attending across the table is a good way to go about it.

My patient was perfect: she'd had some pain episodes, but not severe inflammation or infection. She was between attacks, and her gallbladder was nearly normal. You wouldn't expect to see beautiful robin's-egg blue inside your belly, but that's how the normal gallbladder looks. Gorgeous. It stands out from the earth-tones of everything else in there, like an agate amongst river rocks. It was easily separable in her case from the colon that passes right below it, and the tissues hiding the duct and artery to the gallbladder (called the cystic duct and cystic artery) were soft and manageable. I'd seen it done many times: incise just through the filmy surface layer, tease away the fatty stuff, identify the small duct that connects the gallbladder to the main bile duct. Pass a tie around it, to keep stones from slipping out. Insert a catheter for an X-ray to check the main duct for stones and anatomic aber-rations. Find the artery, tie and cut it. Separate the gallbladder without veering into the liver and making it bleed. Standing to the patient's left, the domain of the assistant, it looks easy. On the right, where the action is, it was like leaning over a cliff: who's back there hanging onto my belt? If you're tremulous when hold-ing very long instruments, they bang against the retractors like an alarm bell, making it very obvious. Afraid to cut too deep. Passing sutures using a long right-angled clamp, around another clamp on the cystic duct, way the hell down there, slipping off, try-ing again. Reaching my index finger far in to cinch the knot, breaking the suture more than once. Every step done over again, coached at first encouragingly then impatiently by the attending. Observing for the first time how important is the exposure pro-vided by the assistant. Noting how much an assistant, who actu-ally knows how to do what you're struggling to figure out, can do with the tip of a suction device. Even closing up was an unex-pected ordeal. How could I have not noticed that the layers of the abdominal wall, whose names I could easily reel off, required more than naming to piece back together? Is that the other edge of the rectus muscle? Where the hell did it go? Unsure at every turn, flailing, I was exhausted at the end, dog-paddling in wet clothes when I'd expected to glide by in Speedos. I was a long way from being in control, from feeling a part of the music that well-performed surgery can be—so far that I didn't even know such a thing existed.

There's a difference between doing surgery and being a surgeon. Some operations are so easy, anyone could do them. With enough bananas, you could teach a chimp to take out an ovary; it's on a stalk, after all, like a mushroom! Cut right here. Place a self-retaining retractor. Put some pads there, and there. Three Kelley clamps. Click, click, and click. Snip, tie, tie, tie. Sew up, slap on a bandage. Next case. Do it again. And again. Pretty soon, it's second nature. I know you could do it.

By the end of the year, I'd removed several gallbladders, and eventually got pretty good at it, cut my time in half. (Some gallbladders are so easy, hanging loosely off the liver—as if on a stalk—that I call them "gynecologic gallbladders.") But I was no surgeon. A surgeon can handle disaster without panicking. He can sort out the anatomy when it isn't as it should be. Calmly stuffing a pack over a bleeding surface and moving deeper, he can find a plane through which to dissect a fat, red, thick, swollen gallbladder off the liver. A surgeon knows when to switch to plan B, or C—and knows that those plans exist. He can come up with plan D when it didn't exist before he invented it. Beyond that, there are good surgeons, and great ones, one of whom was right across town.

eleven

A View of the Master

I got my first look at Victor Richards when I rotated to Children's Hospital, a private hospital loosely associated with UCSF. Not quite sixty, just slightly rotund, Dr. Richards wore a vest under his white coat, draped by a Phi Beta Kappa key. He vibrated with energy, making short humming sounds when he wasn't talking in his tenor voice, as if his own silence were boring him. He spoke several languages (often at the same time), loved theater. Following a precise schedule, he did three cases a day, six days a week, arrived on time, left the hospital by 5:30 every night. His operations always went smoothly and took half the time they would have in the hands of others. Complications, even tiny ones, were so rare as to be like the apocalypse if they occurred. When he made rounds, he avoided retracing his steps: starting on the top floor, he took the front stairs, went down the hall, then the back stairs or fire exit to the lower floor, never passing the nurses' station more than once. Finding efficiency in all things, making everything look easy, he spent only a minute or two in his patients' rooms, but they responded as if they'd been given sacred bones.

Vic Richards had been a Stanford "Whiz Kid." Stanford University did a little human experimentation in the 1920s and 1930s,

identifying several genius children, taking them into an acceler-
ated program, cranking out some precosities. Having earned his
MD at age nineteen, which was too young to get a medical license,
Vic spent some years in the anatomy lab, teaching medical students older than he. He developed his own ideas of how things
were put together and how they came apart, and excelled as a
surgical resident, eventually becoming Chairman of the Stanford
Surgery Department at age thirty. When Stanford moved its hospital facilities from San Francisco to Palo Alto, Vic stayed put and
became one of San Francisco's busiest and best private-practicing
surgeons, sought by the area's richest and most famous, and anyone else who could get in to see him. He had a love-hate relationship with the UCSF professors: they loved to hate him. Despite
his retaining of excellent academic credentials, they didn't see
Vic as one of them; in turn, he spoke of the UCSF professors with
amused and ironic sympathy.

Unless you were a chief resident, spending time at Childrens'
wasn't much of a deal. Vic glommed onto the chief, who left the
junior residents to fend for themselves, assisting and caring for
the patients of the other private docs, most of whom had no desire
to let residents do any part of an operation. It was like the Blue
Service, but without the teaching. There were a few solid surgeons there, along with some cursed to live in surgeon's bodies
but unable to find the control panel. One in particular: a vascular surgeon who divided most of his time between sewing up lacerations in the ER and fixing an occasional hernia tossed to him
when Vic didn't have the time. On the rare occasions he'd actually have a vascular case to do, he'd manage to operate himself
into a corner; then he'd stumble away from the table and beat
his head against the wall, banging away until an idea came loose,

or until he decided to call for help. I didn't know whether to avert my eyes or find him a helmet.

One of the urologists removed kidneys the old-fashioned way: with the patient on his side, going in through the flank (that's not the old part), he'd place a giant clamp under the kidney and across all the vessels at once (that's it). Slice off the kidney, take a huge tie around the combined stump. Most surgeons find each artery and vein and tie them off individually, because if that big clamp slips off, the hole fills up with blood in a hell of a hurry. But he was prepared: a pile of sponges was always at the ready, to be pushed into the hole and leaned on for fifteen minutes while he talked baseball. Which is exactly what happened. The bleeding slowed enough after the fifteen that he could find the vessels and tie them off one by one. Fair enough. But I began to think prevention was better than preparation. It's good to be able to handle problems; best to avoid them.

Oddvar Norqvist was a neurosurgeon, a pleasant man, and possibly nuts. He'd been married to a famous movie star, whose name you'd recognize. Still surgeon to the king of Sweden, he'd occasionally disappear overseas to do things to His Majesty. He'd published a paper on zapping cat brains with diathermy as a way to treat depression. Not having read the paper (he did give me a copy), I can't say how he assessed feline melancholy. But he'd concluded that his machine would work on humans if precisely aimed into the brain, the target determined by calculations from a skull X-ray and dialed into a device attached to the patient's head. This was after anesthetizing the patient and drilling two holes for the probes (I never saw a spaceship but can't say none was involved).

I scrubbed on one case. Before starting, Dr. Norqvist showed me the X-rays, explained in detail how the measurements were taken and translated precisely into the skull device. He spoke to me as if I were a peer, a respected doctor, and for that I always liked him. He drilled the holes, asked for the headgear, and was told it couldn't be found. No problem. As he went to fire up the diathermy machine, he told me to hold the wands in the general direction of the center of the brain. The patient said he felt better the next day. If I thought it would get me the hell out of there, I'd have said it, too.

Oddvar also did back surgery, under local anesthesia. He'd not let an anesthesiologist in the room, nor would he let us order blood to be typed, despite the fact that in most hands, laminectomy (for relieving pressure on the spinal cord and removing a herniated disc) could be bloody. As the nurse would give him his gown, he'd step into it and keep on going, wrapping his arms around her and giving a lingering hug. Sexual assault charges nowadays, but he was such gentle old guy that the nurses just smiled and went on. Positioning the patient on his belly, numbing up the back, he'd cut right down to the bone, chip it away without pain, and spill hardly a drop of blood. It was very impressive. But every patient he admitted for such surgery—without exception—had the same final sentence in his paperwork. "I see no reason for a myelogram [the X-ray that back then was the way to confirm who needed surgery], so often misleading in these cases." I don't know why he was allowed to remain on staff. But his patients went home no worse off than they came in. At Childrens' everyone took it easy; no one made waves. Sort of a gentleman's club. One surgeon had actually been kicked off staff a couple of years earlier but had sued his way back on. Those were different times. Docs still imagined they were in control.

I got a taste of what it was like to scrub with Dr. Richards when he'd have an operation that required an extra pair of hands. He let the chief resident do every one of his cases, but he'd stand to the chief's left, instead of across the table from him like everyone else. Elbowing, cajoling, talking non-stop, reaching in and making a snip, noodling around with his finger, he'd find the target before the chief. Hard to say who was actually doing the operation. Nerve-wracking and intimidating, even humiliating for the chief residents, it was an optional rotation for them, and many avoided it. But at some level I felt a kinship. Not in brilliance, certainly, but in a desire for that efficiency. I sensed that he had an approach to surgery that was different from what we were being taught, and that he was trying in his harassing, vibrating, frenetic way to impart it.

Being a great surgeon is not about having fast hands or making flashy moves. It's about knowing exactly what you want to accomplish, and doing it without wasted motion. Knowing the right thing to do, and doing it right the first time (rarely can a second attempt be executed without exacting a toll on the patient). Anticipating, adjusting. Understanding and being able to find the precise layers and planes between tissues and working within them. Many surgeons don't. I had a teacher in high school, the baseball coach, who liked to say that the best outfielder is the one always making an easy catch. He knows the game situation, watches the catcher set up, sees the signs, figures where he needs to be. You can't avoid all circus catches, but they ought to be rare. Surgery is the same. You admire the surgeon who stops the bleeding, gets out of a tight spot, stays at the bedside in the ICU. I do, too. More, I admire the one who knows how to avoid all that stuff in the first place. A great surgeon makes it look easy. But because the body is resilient, because it will heal itself given half a chance, it mostly doesn't matter. Good enough is good enough. Great is largely wasted. When the bandage goes on, you likely won't be able to tell if your hernia was repaired or your colon resected in a beautiful way, displaying the anatomy cleanly and apposing tissues artfully, or just adequately. You'll be fine either way. But take several hundred patients, or a few really sick ones with no physiologic reserve, and over time you'll see a divergence. Victor Richards was a great surgeon. I wanted to come back as chief resident and see what I could learn.

twelve

A Taste of
the Trauma Team

You can't shine a turd. That was one of Don Trunkey's best-loved
phrases. He'd use it sometimes in the care of an irretrievably failing patient, occasionally in reference to a resident. Don had been
a chief resident when I was an intern, and now, after the two
years I'd been gone, he was on the staff at the County. Big guy,
from eastern Washington cow country, he looked like he ought to
have a straw hat on his head and a blade of grass dangling from
his mouth, saying "Yup" and "Shore thang." Smart, and a good
teacher, his style was to give out a lot of shit, but to do it with a
smile and good humor, so it smelled ok. He loved trauma and
was the attending now, as I rotated back to the County for my
first stint on the trauma team. He's since become one of the
national gurus on the subject, giving lectures on various operative
aspects and being one of the powers behind the trend to desig-
nate hospitals statewide with a particular level of trauma expert-
ise, so that patients are triaged accordingly from the field. The
current interns, and the other first-year residents, knew him only
as staff; to me, he was a friend as well as teacher. There was a
hell of a lot to learn about trauma, and there was some comfort

in knowing that Don had been in my shoes not too long ago, and that his chiding was tempered with understanding. Besides, I generally gave right back—enough that a few years later, a scrub nurse once took me aside, concerned, asking if Dr. Trunkey and I really hated each other. Quite, I told her, the opposite.

Being on the trauma team meant working about a thirty-hour shift, with eighteen hours off, regularly for two months. Since there was rarely time for rest during the shift, time off was spent sleeping or trying to stay awake. Morning rounds were a spectacle. Both teams, plus med students, pharmacists, nurses, various other hangers-on added up to fifteen or twenty people sweeping through the hospital like marauders; lesser men backed away with heads deferentially down. The chief led morning rounds, whose main purpose was to apprise the oncoming team of everything that had gone on the day before, and to make certain that tasks were assigned. Starting in the ICU, we'd go next to the various floors housing our patients, and end in the ER, to see who was still hanging around in the holding wards. Evening rounds were led, unless he was in the OR, by the senior resident. With so many unstable patients, it was essential to round at least twice daily, along with frequent checkups. I kept that up throughout my career; it makes for more efficient care, picks up adverse signs more quickly, gets people well and home sooner.

We spent time on the wards and in the operating room, but the intensive care unit was the center of the vortex for the junior residents. If critical illness were heat, you'd melt in there. Jumping out a sixth-story window does things to a body. So does getting run over by a bus or taking a shotgun to the belly. Having five or six such victims at all times, along with a few lesser recoverees—couple of stab wounds, a bullet or two, ruptured appendix, perforated stomach or colon—produced a broad if wobbly workbench on which to learn to care for the sickest of humanity. Hearts and lungs, kidneys and livers failed alone or in concert, while we dialed in drugs, adjusted the ventilators, calculated fluid and caloric requirements, cleaned wounds, checked drains. With the help of surgical and anesthesia attendings, we became comfortable juggling disparate needs of multiple patients, street performers in white coats. *Cirque du malaise.*

It mystifies me how frequently San Francisco MUNI buses managed to run people down. Maybe it's the fog. We saw such crunches regularly. Even had a patient who got hit and survived multiple organ injuries and a two-month hospitalization; got hit again on the day of discharge, as he used the crosswalk in front of the hospital, heading to the bus stop across the street.

Darwin might have been wrong: when you see the body's response to massive trauma, you have to figure that evolution bailed out early. If you get yourself into that kind of mess, it said, you're gonna die. Up to a point, shock is a reasonable response to injury. First of all, it makes you lie down, if you're not smart enough to do it yourself. Then it shuts off the blood going to unimportant places—your arms and legs and belly, for example—and sends it where it's most needed: your brain and heart. But since you'd like to have your kidneys, your liver, and your bowels back at some point, you'll want to return circulation to those places before too long. For small injuries (maybe the things evolution was dealing with) it works out fine—lie down, have a bowl of mastodon soup. But for major modern trauma, body response can become disease, with treatment making it worse. Injury releases various bad substances into the bloodstream which can make capillaries leaky (the smallest and most diffuse and metabolically active blood vessels). So when you give the huge amounts of fluids needed to overcome deep shock, it seeps out everywhere.

Cutting Remarks

The body becomes one of those party-favor sponges that quadruple in size when you add water, turning itself into an unrecognizable shiny-skinned blob; worse, the lungs fill up with fluids. Patients need ventilators, using higher and higher pressures to hammer air through the soup in their chest. Then the high pressure and high oxygen levels themselves cause more problems: perforated lungs, oxygen toxicity. Or this: injury makes blood more likely to clot, which makes good sense. But it can go crazily wrong, making little clots form throughout the bloodstream, which eats up all the protein factors needed for blood to clot, which then causes uncontrollable bleeding everywhere. These conditions—ARDS (acute respiratory distress syndrome) and DIC (disseminated intravascular coagulation)—end in death for many badly injured patients. Dr. Blaisdell, and Trunkey and others after him, made several important contributions to their treatment. At the County we were witness to, and participants in, the occasional save of the previously unsalvageable; and after doing it for days on end, some of it sinks in.

A couple of interesting paradoxes: protein in the bloodstream is what keeps the liquid part of blood where it belongs, in the vessels (exerting what's called "oncotic pressure"). What Blazer showed is that giving albumin (the critical protein) to prevent leaking and ARDS, as was advocated in lots of places, made things worse. And he showed that to stop the bleeding of DIC, you give anticoagulants (blood thinners).

Tending the wards, out of the ICU, was like being some sort of deviant gardener. Working our way up and down rows of beds lined along the edges of narrow, cavernous rooms, separated by curtains which hung like under-watered foliage—drooping, dirty, shredded—we cultivated patients who were in various states of mute acceptance or vocal defiance. "This pain medicine you're givin' me ain't fer shit" was the most common salutation. (Until, after a day or two of complaining, they'd be pleasantly compliant on morning rounds, having made the connection; the night shift orderlies had a side business going. Drugs flowed when the lights went out.) The open wards, while highly efficient, by definition prevented intimacy, exacerbating an already precarious relationship. No one was happy to be there; most had fallen victim to their own or someone else's stupidity or violence. Some were in withdrawal from alcohol or drugs; many weren't anxious to return to their home life, while we were trying to get them well and out of there. Gratitude was not in the air. But I loved it. This was a real county hospital, the ferment of its wards connecting back to the earliest days of hospitals in this country, and across the seas to Europe. I felt it every time I entered.

The prison ward, on the other hand, was just creepy. It was an open area too, but you passed through locked doors to get in, there were guards with guns, and scary patients. Guys shot by cops, drug dealers who made the wrong deal. My skin felt prickly there. Once, while changing a bandage, the news came on the one TV in the middle of the room, talking about this very person, a double murderer, shot while attempting escape. Seeing his face on the screen and in front of me, I might have made a cute remark, had he not looked at me with an expression that burns even today: got something you wanna say, motherfucker?

I didn't do much in the OR as junior trauma resident: most time was spent in patient care. Got to take out the occasional appendix, sometimes do a low-suspicion abdominal exploration. The rectum, however, was my undisputed free-fire zone. In San Francisco, it was not a rarity to be called upon to remove a foreign object from someone's hindmost. The chief residents' room had a collection of several, tastefully displayed. An attempt would be made to dislodge the item in the ER, but because of discomfort, it wasn't often possible. (There was one successful ER extraction while I was in the Mish, and the results were posted proudly on a bulletin board: the object had been sent to the pathology lab, and the report was there for all to see. "Normal cucumber, with feces.") So we'd take those patients to the OR, give them a spinal, and pull the object out, usually after the dust had settled on everything else around three a.m. Candles, dildoes, a highly-polished hatchet handle, a maraschino cherry jar. A fluorescent bulb. In one such wee-hour escapade, I removed a vibrator and brought it to the head of the table.

"Here it is, Mr. Jones. What would you like us to do with it?"

"Oh, how about changing the batteries and putting it back in?"

thirteen

Gut and Glory

Dr. Dunphy liked to scrub at least once with each of his second-year residents. The stars had to align just right: he was away a lot, and appropriate cases didn't come up on command. When it worked out, it could be the only chance you'd get, and it had the aura of a pass-fail test to make it into the senior years. Our case was a right colon resection, for cancer. I thought it might be a bad sign when he scrubbed in and called me Schwartz.

When you're still an embryo, your intestines are floating out in front of you, and your belly is wide open. As development proceeds, the intestines corkscrew their way inside, and the colon lays itself down around the inner periphery of your abdomen, in the shape of an inverted horseshoe. The right ("ascending") colon is the first part, beginning where the small intestine joins it, in the lower right part of your belly. It heads up the right side to the liver, takes a left turn and crosses under your stomach (becoming the "transverse colon"), heads up toward the spleen (the "splenic flexure"), makes a hairpin turn down to the left side (the left, or "descending" colon), and finally takes an S-shaped ("sigmoid" colon) spin into the rectum. The blood vessels to the colon head outward from the middle of your belly, like hands on a clock. All of that derives from the embryological corkscrew, and it means that if you cut it loose from its outside attachments to the abdominal wall, you can deliver the colon up into your hands where you can work on it quite easily (unless it's stuck and swollen from infection or a large tumor, or has perforated and retracted inward, or any of a number of other things that can make it anything but easy). Doing that—separating the colon from the sides of the abdominal wall—has always struck me as one of the neatest things a surgeon does. It's like knowing one of the body's deepest secrets: this big long fat bloody tube, which seems tightly stuck in there, can in fact, with the most delicate of maneuvers, be made to lift right out while still connected to its blood vessels. The trick is inserting your hand in just the right place laterally and doing a "c'mere" motion with your first two or three fingers, then cutting the thinned-out layer you've made. It's nearly bloodless up the right side and down the left (it does get harder in between).

That's what Dr. Dunphy was trying to get me to do but, being a colonic virgin, I was bashful. I'd had a chance to put a few stitches in bowel, do part of an anastomosis (putting the cut ends back together) in past operations, but never had I done it from start to finish. "If you can see through it, you can cut it," he said. That, it turns out, is the single most useful thing I ever heard from him— other than several good jokes. It seems pretty obvious, and I guess it is. But it's really helpful to remember when doing a difficult dissection in an area where all normal anatomy has been distorted or obliterated. Still, I was afraid of starting bleeding, of puncturing the colon, of being surprised by the duodenum (a portion of which hides back there, intimidating and daring you to touch it). Nor was it any easier doing the rest of it: selecting the place to divide the colon, clearing it of fat down to the surface. Finding, securing, and dividing the feeding blood vessels. Is it fat in here, or is it just me? "What are you going to do next?" he'd ask. "Here, let me show you," if I didn't get to it quickly enough.

Sewing bowel together feels to me like a connection across centuries to the surgeons who first braved it. Today you can use staplers, and in some situations they make a very positive difference. But recently trained surgeons use them for every hookup, and I think that's a big mistake. Any time saved (none, in most cases—plus they are huge chunks of plastic and steel that get tossed after a single use) is more than offset by enormous added cost; nor does it make it safer. But mostly, by using those staplers, they're missing out on one of the most satisfying things we do. An artfully made bowel anastomosis is a thing of beauty. There's an inner row of dissolving suture, in a running fashion, from the back side to the front, done in such a way as to make it all turn inward, and an outer row of individual (interrupted) stitches, requiring turning the tip of the needle holder in a perfectly circular motion, digging the exact depth to penetrate the outer surface and muscle, but not the inner layer (mucosa). As you watch the edges disappear inward, and see a row of evenly spaced sutures complete a perfect circle, no mucosa showing; as you observe the tiny nearby arteries dancing their proof that you haven't disrupted the blood supply to the edges, you know you can safely drop it back inside, a secret gift to the patient. Of course, I was years from being artful and I've always assumed Dr. Dunphy was not impressed. But he didn't fire me.

Bruised egos need love. Not long after the colon procedure, I was scrubbing with Tom Hunt on a jejuno-ileal bypass—one of the first operations widely done for weight loss in the massively obese; it worked by causing diarrhea and malabsorption. There are much better choices now, and j-i bypass has been abandoned.

Cutting Remarks

But at the time Dr. Hunt was interested in them and did quite a few. It was a wide-open operation, and in large people, exposing the operative field was tough work. We found ourselves each with one hand holding fat and bowel out of the way; with his other hand Tom had placed a suture in the intestine. The stitch needed tying, but neither of us could

Dr Hunt was more scholarly than the average surgeon. Friendly but distant, in the way that comes from having ten thoughts in your brain at once, he gave the impression of always being spaced-out. He asked a patient if she liked the food, ignoring the stomach tube dangling from her nose. He was also one of the interviewers I had, seeking internship. Wonder if he was paying attention.

release our exposure-providing hand. While he stood there looking at it for a moment, I had a flash: we could each use a free hand to double-team it. He held one end of the suture while I threw a one-handed knot and cinched it down, then I held the other end while he did the same. Tom had been around a long time but that was a new one. He was impressed, even suggested I write it up for a "How I Do It" section of a surgical journal (someone actually did, many years later). Not exactly a cure for cancer, it nevertheless made me think my brain was not completely devoid of surgical wiring.

fourteen

Pus and Burns

A highlight of the second year of residency was the SFGH Pus
Service, officially known by the less descriptive term, Extremity
Service. By definition a collection of arm and leg problems, it
dealt primarily with infections, which meant draining abscesses
caused by shooting up infected heroin. Rectal abscesses, though
hardly part of an extremity, were also on the list. In one of my
more humiliating moments, I took a man to the OR in the middle of the night for what clearly must have been such an abscess,
but after probing for too long, couldn't find a collection to drain.
"Hey, everyone," the nurse said. "Schwab's doing a white-owl
butt case." Took him back the next morning, with the attending,
who found it with difficulty, high up.

The service consisted of a second-year resident and an intern,
so the resident was, in effect, a chief resident, even giving a report
at the D and C conference. When I was in high school, I worked
on a grounds crew for the school district. During my second year,
they let me drive my own truck with a younger kid in my charge.
Wearing a hard hat, and scrunching my arm against the window
sill of the truck so it looked like I had big biceps, I'd drive around
smoking cigars, feeling much cooler than I was. That's what it
was like being chief of the Pus Service.

Not that draining pus is inconsequential: way back in med school, I'd learned that. But, heartless residents that we were, what we craved was the occasional suicide attempt wherein the wrists were slashed, deep enough to do some damage. Then we called Gene Kilgore, a world-renowned hand surgeon, who would come over from his downtown practice and talk us through the repair. Using suture fine as hair, beautifully delicate instruments, and double-headed operating microscopes, we found and reapproximated ends of nerves, making precise movements, suturing and tying with metallic jaws so small you could make a watch with them, each action magnified. Tremors looked like tidal waves. Tendons were put together with clever U-shaped stitches, like embroidery. It was great fun. One such repair was the only time Judy has ever seen me operate; I brought her into the OR late one night. Nobody cared.

But pus was our mission, so when Eric Austin showed up, I made ready for a typical drainage procedure. And watched him nearly die.

There were ORs at the County that were another trip back in time: the kind with tile walls and unenclosed bleachers where students used to sit and watch as the professor, likely dressed in a suit under his rubber apron, lectured and operated barehanded. In the early 1900s, so it's said, Leo Eloesser—a pioneer chest surgeon for whom various operations are named—operated thusly on the Ambassador from Spain, removing a lung for cancer. When he stopped to write on a chalkboard, demonstrating, the clamp slipped off, and the man bled to death instantly. Eloesser kept right on talking, rolled His Excellency over, and proceeded with an autopsy. Those were the very rooms in which we now sat for lectures, and I heard the echoes. Even the main operating rooms had observer access from the floor above: once a drunken visitor somehow found his way into the gallery, sat down, and watched as we worked on a gunshot victim.

You've heard of it as "flesh-eating disease." The proper term is necrotizing fasciitis ("NEH-cruh-tie-zing fash-ee-EYE-tiss"), meaning an infection that destroys the tough layer (fascia) surrounding muscles, and sometimes the muscles themselves. When the press hears about a case, they tend to give it breathless coverage; but it's been around forever, and you can't catch it from someone who has it. What's required is the perfectly wrong combination of injury and a couple of species of bacteria that aid each other's growth while producing gas, which bubbles through the tissues and moves the infection along at a frightening rate. You can feel the gas; it's like a layer of teeny bubble-wrap, popping under your fingers as you examine the area. Unlike the patient with a simple abscess or uncomplicated tissue infection (cellulitis), these people can look sick as hell. Thready pulse, flushed and fevered, maybe a bit incoherent. Put a mark on the edge of the red zone, and a few minutes later you see the redness has moved an inch or two. If you still can't figure out what's going on, take an X-ray and see the gas staring back at you. It's a horrible thing.

Eric Austin had played softball in Golden Gate Park, taking a knee to his thigh as he slid into second base. By that evening, it hurt too much to walk, so he lay on his couch for a couple of days until he started to feel ill, at which point he called a friend who brought him to the Mission. When you see necrotizing fasciitis, usually there's an entry point of broken skin, or the patient is a diabetic or otherwise compromised. Eric was healthy and intact, and given his story, it wasn't surprising that there was no urgency in the call I got to see him in the ER. It figured to be your basic infected blood clot, needing routine "I and D" (incision and drainage). He was in pain, and his thigh was red and swollen, but I wasn't alarmed until I put my hand on him and felt the crepitus (the crunch of tissue-air). Then, for the first of countless times in my career, I called the OR and said I had someone who needed a room ASAP; and I called my attending.

You expect fat to be bright yellow, and to bleed a bit as you cut through it. When it's gray and fizzes, it makes you sick to your stomach. It's even worse when muscle and fascia look that way. The only cure for necrotizing fasciitis is to remove all the involved tissues and give big doses of antibiotics. And go back to the OR once, twice, as often as it takes, to do it all again. Even when you think you've gotten ahead of the advancing line, you may not have. We cut away most of the muscles of Eric's thigh, front and back, and the skin over them. It looked impossible to save his leg, but at that point we'd removed everything that looked infected; and since I hadn't thought to discuss amputation with him, we took him to the ICU to wake him up and talk things over before the next operation. He was lucid, and adamant: no amputation. He'd rather die, he said, than lose his leg. I was as clear and as insistent as I could be. So was he. When his pulse and temperature began to rise, we took him back to the OR.

Dr. Blaisdell was not the official attending, but he'd heard about the case and preempted his way in. Within minutes it became obvious: there was no way to save Eric's leg, and it didn't look like we'd save his life. The infection now involved the remaining muscles of his leg, had worked its way into the buttocks, and worst of all, the fascia of the psoas muscle—which goes way up the back side of the belly, behind the kidney and beyond.

"He needs disarticulation," Blazer said, meaning taking the whole leg including the hip joint. It's the worst kind of amputation from which to re-hab, because without a stump there's no control over any prosthesis you'd fashion.

"Dr. Blaisdell," I said, "he was as clear as he could be: he refuses amputation. He says he'd rather die."

"He's septic [the effects of infection in the bloodstream]. I'll testify that he's mentally impaired if I have to. No twenty-year-old is going to die here for lack of an amputation," Blazer said. Forcefully.

"Really," I offered, by now not at all sure what was right. "He was very clear."

"Then I'll do it."

So I did it. And more. When we were done, his hip socket was empty, his buttocks were denuded all around to the middle of his back, his lower belly had no skin either, and his left testicle was hanging in the breeze like an Easter egg on a string. We'd reached up behind his abdomen and uncovered the psoas as far as we could, and left a bunch of rubber drains. It was going to be hard to face him when he awoke, as certain as he'd been about what he wanted. On the other hand, I was sure he was going to die.

Dr. Blaisdell was just leaving the ICU when I got there at 5:30 the next morning. That was uncomfortable enough, but he said, "Your patient just wrote a note. You better go read it." (He was still on a ventilator and couldn't talk.) Call my lawyer, was what I expected, and my stomach hurt as I looked at the clipboard. "I'd like information on prostheses, please" is what it said.

Eric never mentioned his pre-op declaration. Blazer was right; he didn't even remember it. (Raises interesting questions about "informed consent" in the face of critical illness, doesn't it?) After another couple of operations to tidy up, he was clearly a survivor. To keep his broad areas of denuded muscle clean, I sweet-talked the night shift nurses in the burn unit into helping me use the brand-new Hubbard tank, in a room down the hall: a stainless-steel high-power whirlpool designed with burn patients in mind. Trouble was, no one on the night shift knew how to use it. We guessed at how much soap to use, lowered him in, and cranked the tank. Bad guess. The tank turned into a frothy overflowing roil, a soapy wave sweeping across the room. Ironic if we cured the bad bubbles, and the good ones drowned him. We bailed with our hands and with buckets, washing the foam down the sinks. Eric was amused. The folks in X-ray, one floor below, were not. In a frenzy, they called asking what the hell was going on up there—their toilets and sinks overflowing, equipment shutting down. Hmm. No idea, I told them. No one ratted on me, but we didn't use the tank again. After skin grafting and some rehab, Eric was discharged, after I left the service. I'd love to know what became of him.

When I had first come onto the Extremity Service, I inherited a similar patient. Jose Castro was an addict who'd infected his left arm while shooting up. He'd developed fasciitis, but the muscles weren't involved, so he'd had all the skin of his arm and shoulder removed, front and back, along with the fascia covering the muscles. Having no skin from his wrist to his neck, to the middle of his chest and back down to his waist, he looked like page two of the textbook on anatomy of the shoulder. He'd survived many episodes of septic shock before my time and now was undergoing twice-daily dressing changes to cleanse his muscles before applying skin grafts. Hell of a tough guy: he was determined never again to use narcotics, and insisted we do our work without any medications. We'd peel away the previous bandages—rolls of antiseptic-soaked gauze—exposing each muscle group, while his hand and arm were suspended from an IV pole. He must have been monstrous at one time: even after his long illness he looked like Mr. Universe, and his muscles glistened like marble. A

Michelangelo. Jose's face reddened, beads of sweat formed on his brow, but he produced a smile over a tight jaw as we worked. I got most of Jose's grafting done before I left the service, and he went home a few weeks later. Next year he got loaded, fell down some stairs, and died of a head injury, back at the County.

✳

The reason I knew the burn unit nurses when we sloshed Eric Austin is that burns were the responsibility of the Pus Service. That's a strange combination, since infection is what ultimately does in the fatal burn victims. We washed like hell and wore sterile gowns whenever we went in. Washed like hell, entered hell. A burn unit is one of the worst places on Earth.

Sunburn is a first-degree burn; blistering is second-degree. With third-degree the skin is destroyed. (There's fourth-degree, too: burned muscle, tendons, bone. Think of that: burned bone. Awful.) Take the percent of the body burned to the third degree, add the victim's age, and you have an estimate of the chance of dying. Alex Williams had a ninety-percent third-degree burn, and he was eighteen years old. He'd been in there several weeks, surviving against the odds. Someone had tossed a Molotov cocktail into his garage while he was working—apparently not at random. The top of his head was the only area spared.

Burn away skin and you open a direct line for bacteria into the bloodstream. Treatment aims at getting coverage as quickly as possible, ideally with the patient's own skin, grafted from somewhere else. (It's a "split-thickness" graft: you shave off just the outermost layer , leaving much of the skin in place. When it grows a new surface, you can do it again. There are other options: pig skin, cadaver skin.) First, you have to get rid of the burned part.

It may be possible to cut it all away at once, in the OR, and immediately place a skin graft or skin substitute. But when it's a really extensive burn, it can become a matter of slathering on bactericidal creams and bandages, changing them frequently, and picking away dead tissue bit by bit, allowing granulation tissue to form in its place, making a base for grafting. That's what nurses in the burn unit do, often to the screams of their patients. To watch them do it is to see two people brutalized. Nurses there burn out (no joke) more rapidly than in any other part of a hospital; it's against their nature to inflict pain. For months they'd done a magnificent and excruciating job with Alex Williams and were like grizzlies with a cub. I was an intruder.

A second-year resident knows a few things about a few things, but I made no pretense of knowing burns. The nurses knew plenty and had very strong opinions of what ought to happen. Don Trunkey was the permanent attending in charge of the burn unit; they listened to and trusted him. Us too-young residents—we were barely tolerated. At least I was smart enough to recognize my place: I asked for their suggestions, and kept otherwise out of their way. I was there to learn from Don and from the nurses.

Alex was defying the odds, but he hadn't beaten them. We, and those before us, shaved skin from his scalp as often as possible to get another small area covered, and we used pig skin. Going first for his hands and face, we were still dealing with an enormous expanse of raw surface; Alex had had many episodes of sepsis, which were becoming more frequent, more resistant to antibiotics. He was a heartbreakingly cooperative and trusting kid; you could see it in what was left of his face. He'd come this far as much by force of his own determination as by the care he was getting, but there was another problem. The metabolic requirements of a burn victim can be staggering, and Alex wasn't getting anywhere near enough calories: he developed diarrhea if we pushed tube-feeding too hard, and he was getting maximum levels of intravenous feedings. With each septic episode he lost more kidney function, became less arousable. It became obvious that he was finally going to die, and that the nurses were going to be devastated and angry. When the time came, it was worse than I imagined, preceded by a decision—with which some of the nurses disagreed—to stop the antibiotics and give pain meds only. I'd talked it over for days with Don. Alex's family accepted the truth, painfully. But as the person who wrote the orders, I was looked at through icy eyes. I understood, I felt terrible, but I also resented it, since I'd simply been the one there for the immutable ending. Don met with the nurses several times: group therapy for a horrible and unprecedented situation. We ended up on acceptable terms, and there were some routine patients that came and went in routine ways. But I was glad when it was over.

fifteen

Loose Ends of the Second Year, and a Vision

When I returned to the Vascular Service as a junior resident, I watched the destruction of two human beings in a single moment. I was assisting on a particularly difficult carotid endarterectomy, wherein the artery is opened and obstructing cholesterol desposits (called plaques) are cleaned out through an incision in the artery, made between clamps to prevent bleeding. The plaques usually are demarcated and limited to the crotch between major branches; in this case, it was tailing much higher than usual, requiring an extra-long incision, and placing the upper clamp in an awkward way. The surgeon had an intern steadying the clamp. Time is critical: the longer the operation takes, the greater the risk of stroke. Some surgeons were beginning to use plastic shunts to supply blood around the clamps, but this attending didn't believe in them. As the work dragged on, he got more and more agitated. Shunts are routine now; such a thing wouldn't happen today. Meanwhile, having been pushed further and further away as the operator got more and more frustrated, the intern was holding the clamp nearly at arm's length, unable to see what he was doing, nor to feel the strain on the clamp, until, with a sickening pop, the carotid was levered right out of the patient's skull, like a cork out of a wine-bottle. I don't know if that's ever happened before or since, but with the end retracted back above bone, there was no way to fix it, or even to control the bleeding. The surgeon glared at the intern, shaking and reddening, and, as only a surgeon can do, affixed blame: "You just killed my patient."

Remembering well my experience with Gary Davis, I sought out the intern and tried to console him. "It wasn't your fault," I said. "The surgeon is in charge, and he was literally pushing you away. He should have known. There was nothing you could have done differently." I tried for an hour, but the intern was inconsolable. Devastated. A very bright and sensitive young man—maybe too much so to be a surgeon—he couldn't face the vascular attendings again, and left the internship that day. He got a job at a hospital across the Bay but, I was told, left medicine altogether at the end of the year.

The best thing about being back on vascular was operating again with Jerry Goldstone, who was now a vascular fellow, and later became an attending in the department. (He'd also become a good friend. When there was mutual time, he and Linda and Judy and I went to any of several favorite restaurants.) There aren't a lot of vascular operations lowly enough to hand down. One was sympathectomy, a last-ditch operation. The sympathetic nerves are part of the autonomic nervous system and lie along the spine. To dilate leg arteries, you head to the belly, making an incision in the abdominal wall, right at the level of the belly-button, and working your way to the spine without ever getting inside the abdominal cavity. Sounds like magic, like the saw-a-lady-in-half trick. Jerry showed me how. And if you develop kidney failure, I could make a connection between an artery and vein in your wrist for hooking you up to a kidney machine. They let me do that too.

I also was on TV. The American College of Surgeons met every three years in San Francisco, and part of the deal was televising live operations to an auditorium downtown, where surgeons watched and could ask questions of the ones doing the work. It had become legendary: closed-circuit TV activates surgical poltergeists. A broken femur (thigh bone) was rodded; when the drapes came off, the foot was rotated ninety degrees. A colon polyp was searched for and never found. Demonstrating repair of a hernia under local anesthesia, the surgeon had to contend with a patient who was jumping all over the place. These things had happened, according to legend, in past broadcasts. (The live operations are no longer part of the meeting. It's not hard to figure why.) On this occasion, I was helping Jerry do a porta-caval shunt—making a connection between the vena cava ("Big Blue," the main vein carrying blood to the heart from the torso) and the portal vein (taking blood from the gut to the liver). It's done to relieve pressure in the hemorrhage-prone veins around the stomach and esophagus caused by cirrhosis of the liver. It can be tough, because before the shunt is completed and the pressure is lowered, blood bubbles up from everywhere, like an incoming tide. The plan was to get all the anatomy laid out before we went live, and spend the air time doing the venous anastomosis. Five minutes before going on, when we were almost there, we got into some bleeding from the pancreas and spent the whole show getting it stopped, Jerry taking crap from the amused audience. I wrote "Hi Mom" on the knuckles of my glove with a surgical marking pen, and hung on to the retractors, my hand a

comforting backdrop to Jerry's struggle. We finished after we
went off air.

The year ended with three single-month rotations away from
general surgery. First was another stint on transplant. More of
the same, except that I got to plug in a couple of kidneys. It was
good experience in sewing vessels and repairing bladders. Only
a few liver transplants had been done in the world, mostly in
Denver. I was there for the first one in the UCSF series, which
turned out badly. You can't remove a failed transplant and put
the patient on a liver machine.

There was a second spin on orthopedics, this time at the County,
getting handy at drilling pins through the shinbone, setting up
pulleys and weights to attach to the pin, providing traction for a
broken femur. That was fun, but you'll hardly see it nowadays;
femur fractures are rodded internally, right down the inner shaft
of the bone, and it works a hell of a lot better (except when it's
done on TV). I saw other workings of the orthopedic mind: wanting to avoid talking to their patients more than once, the orthopedic residents pushed the cart full of charts to the far end of the
ward, then zig-zagged their way back up the rows to round on
their patients. Innovative. If you see patients by going down along
one wall and back up the other, the ones in the first row have
time to think of questions by the time you pass again. The chief
resident looked like she'd stepped out of a centerfold into her
scrubs. Tougher than any man, a year later she had a baby the
day after doing a big operation. She eventually became department head, and a few years later got notoriety advocating invol-
untary AIDS testing on patients. No doctor in the country was

more at risk for getting AIDS than an orthopedist at San Francisco General Hospital: drills and saws turning bone marrow into an aerosol several times a day, floating into their faces.

✳

Esoteric and tedious, neurosurgery impressed but didn't attract me. Charlie Wilson, however, amazed me. Chairman of the department, he radiated enough energy to power the place had the lights gone out. A marathon runner before it became widespread, he spent the rest of his time at the hospital, all hours, day and night. He was a superb operator, tackling brain tumors others refused, getting results far better than expected. He looked you right in the eye, drilling the truth in deep, exuding understated confidence. Patients came from all over the world, handing him their brains.

One of the neurosurgeons looked like an alien, come to Earth to help us, if allowed to breathe methane. He did all his cases with a self-designed, fully enclosed mask, dangling two exhaust hoses over his shoulders and down his back. As he meticulously attended to bleeding, one corpuscle at a time, his operations took hours longer than anyone else's. But they said he'd never had a post-op hematoma (blood collection), never an infection. Of course not: any bacterium that wandered into the wound would have died of boredom or starved to death.

In a world where looks matter, kids with craniofacial abnormalities are screwed. When their facial bones and sections of skull fuse prematurely, or grow in the wrong direction, some are so disfigured you want to look away. A French surgeon, Paul Tessier, had developed a spectacular and wondrous approach to such problems, doing operations that lasted twelve hours and longer— unroofing the entire top of the skull, cutting out cubes of bone containing the eyeballs, moving them outward, rearranging entire sections of facial aberration that formerly had been set in stone. One of the neurosurgeons at UC had gone to Paris to study with Tessier and brought him back to San Francisco to put on a clinic. I didn't have the time to watch an entire operation, but what I saw has stayed with me.

Dr. Tessier brought his team with him: an anesthetist, a tech, and a scrub nurse. It was the *pas de deux* performed by Tessier and his nurse that opened my eyes and dropped my jaw. As he sat, focused like a cat on his work, he'd raise a hand wordlessly and his nurse would give him an instrument, which he'd bring to the field, work for a moment, then pass it back and receive another one. Never a hesitation, never a wrong move, it flowed like a ballet, musically, the noblest art humans can create among themselves. Still clumsy, I could nevertheless recognize perfection. That, I thought, is what it can be, what it *must* be to do surgery.

It's a rarity. Few surgeons get to do the same thing over and over, in the same place, with the same team. Instead, it's night shift, day shift, one hospital, two or three. You try to find the rhythm, to get a flow going, with you, your assistant, your scrub nurse all knowing what's coming, facilitating, cooperating. In a tough spot, you want to maintain focus, not moving your head, keeping the area you've just exposed perfectly in view. Hand out, wanting the right tool slapped in smartly, you don't want to fumble for it, nor lose sight, nor have to reposition the instrument; boring in, you try to keep it going, saying, "I'll be using a long Allis next." But instead of getting it you hear, "Sue, can you get me a long Allis from central supply?" "Geez! This is a low pelvic case. I always use a long Allis." "Sorry doctor. I usually scrub ortho." Screech. Nureyev drops Fonteyn on her ass.

I'll divert to the present long enough to say that in my practice I got close. My clinic hired away the hospital's best scrub nurse, Joanie Thompson, and I worked with her on most of my cases. When I did, we were a hell of a team. She knew. She always had what I needed. When I'd want an instrument different from what I typically used, Joanie had it before I asked. "I'll need a longer needle holder, and mount it backwards." Whack, into my hand, the suture perfectly placed in the jaws. "And make it snappy," I'd say, after the fact. The pleasure from an operation allowed to flow, where every step follows logically from the last, where each move is fluid without stops and diversions, is transcendent. It restores the soul. It makes you want to sing, which I often did. Joanie told me the best thing I ever heard as a surgeon: "You make this look so easy," she said. She became an RNFA (Registered Nurse First Assistant)—in fact, she's a national force in making that occupation a reality; she's just as good an assistant as she was a scrub. But I always missed having Joanie pop an instrument into my hand, the right one, at the right time, making music.

Toward the end of the second year, the dance begins: who gets to finish training, who goes? Lab year? Two? I looked at a couple of lab positions; I considered working with Larry Way at the VA, in his biliary research lab. Academic surgery was not my aim, but extra work operating on bile ducts might be fun. Except that it was on monkeys. When I checked out the lab, they were strapped into modified high chairs: tubes coming out of their bellies, trays keeping their hands and feet away. Sitting there endlessly, staring without expression, wondering why. I'm no antivivisectionist, but that I couldn't do.

Maybe the profs in charge took pity on me since I was already a year or two behind because of my military service. I was given a chance to skip the lab year and go directly to a senior resident slot. If nothing else, the lab year was a time to digest, to go to conferences, to let it all sink in. I wondered if I'd learned enough to be ready. But I figured someone must think I'd be ok. I took it.

part

The Beginning

three

sixteen

Senior Resident
at the County

Night and day doesn't do it. Sea and shore? Earth and moon? Baseball and whipped cream. It's hard doing justice to the difference between a junior and a senior resident, and to how surprised I was that it fit so well. Those first three years, it turns out, were less about building skills than about gaining judgment. Seeing situation after situation, witnessing all manner of mayhem and mastery, cramming three normal work-weeks into one, month after month—darned if some of it hadn't found its way into my gray matter, making connections. I'd been so concerned over what I hadn't yet learned about doing surgery that I'd not noticed how much I'd picked up about being a surgeon. It's good that I had because a senior resident on trauma is a roving surgical consultant. When the medical docs needed a surgeon, I got the call.

There was, in training, an uneasy relationship between surgeons and internists. Competitive rather than

I don't know what they called us. We called them "fleas," as in hopping around and annoying. Especially in the ICU, which was a sort of joint venture among specialties, they felt the need to make comments and suggestions, which we felt the need to ignore. There wasn't much they had to offer that we thought we couldn't handle ourselves. Youthful delusion, to a large extent.

cooperative, it stemmed from many issues, not the least of which, I think, was our less than fully formed confidence in ourselves. Nor, as different as the two callings are, is it surprising that each would see the other as somehow deficient. Internists think surgeons are just technicians—thoughtless cutters who'd operate on anyone or anything unless reined in. To a surgeon, an internist is someone who talks all day and gets very little accomplished. We understood medical issues; they were clueless about surgery. One of the many pleasures of finishing training and entering the real world was the discovery of how wrong all that stuff was, and how much better patient care is served by a collegial attitude among doctors. Not only is it better; it's one of the greatest pleasures of private practice.

You'd think that in a place with surgeons on staff as talented as Blaisdell and Trunkey (and several others whom I've not mentioned) there'd be a high level of trust by the medical types, and that certain truths would not have to be learned over and over. Such as: when a GI bleeder has received more than six or eight pints of blood in a short time, there gets to be a vicious cycle; if most of the blood in your veins belongs to someone else, it doesn't work well. For one thing, it doesn't clot anymore. A GI bleeder who has lost several units faces steadily lowering odds of stopping non-surgically. Yet when someone with massive bleeding was admitted to the medical service, he'd be hidden from the surgeons for as long as possible. Surgeons kill people, the senior medical residents told their juniors. Send them a hemorrhaging patient, they'll operate and send him back dead. So they'd pour in more and more blood, flush the stomach with ice water, dance their dance around the bed until the patient was in profound shock, making no urine, bleeding from everywhere. Then they'd call for a surgical consult. And with no other choice, we'd operate. Sure enough, the patient would die. And the medical docs would say amongst themselves, "See? Told ya."

Some of the GI fellows (internists taking extra training—"Fellowship"—in intestinal diseases) were different. They saw value in surgeons and believed in keeping them informed. (It's natural: the more you hang around surgeons, the more you like them.) If such a fellow were involved, I'd get a call for a consult early in the process. Once, it was about a man admitted with steady but not brisk upper GI bleeding. He'd been scoped and found to have diffuse gastritis; the whole inner lining of his stomach was oozing. Imagine taking sandpaper to your forearm, rubbing beyond the pain until it's red and raw and dripping blood: it's like that. The surgical options aren't good; you can't suture the entire gastric lining. There's vagotomy—which has no more than a toss-up chance of working—or, in desperate cases, removing all or most of the stomach. Not a situation you want to be in. When I saw the patient, he was bleeding pleasantly enough: easy to keep up with, but showing no sign of slowing. I remember a puzzled and worried look on his face, no panic. Waiting, working to maintain calm; when are you guys going to do something? His routine clotting tests were normal, but I found he'd been taking aspirin, which sticks to platelets (an important component of blood clotting) and makes them stop working. Giving fresh

The medical options aren't magic either. Correct bleeding abnormalities, do something about stomach acid. They also liked to irrigate the stomach with ice water, on the theory that it makes blood vessels constrict. That drove Blazer crazy: he'd done studies that show cold inactivates clotting proteins. He'd point out that barbers put a hot towel on your face for those little oozers after a shave. On the trauma service, we used warm water. How weird is that: entirely different approaches at opposite ends of the same hospital?

platelets can correct the problem, but the lab doc refused to release them, because the patient's total platelet count was normal.

I went down to the lab and talked directly to the doc, pointing out that the total number of platelets made no difference if they were ineffective. Even went back and personally tested bleeding time, which is a way to check platelet function, and it was abnormally long. Still the labfuhrer fixated on the total count, and stood fast. It's hard to explain what an idiotic position that was: like saying because there's more water outside than inside, your boat isn't sinking. To give platelets at the County, you needed permission from the lab doc. But because the trauma team ruled, and more importantly because Dr. Blaisdell was an expert in blood-clotting issues, we—and only we—could give them without permission. But only to our own patients. So, after talking the medical docs into it, I transferred the patient to the trauma service, at which point all I had to do was write the order. Done, and done, and the bleeding stopped. When I transferred him back, there was no need to say anything, but my thoughts were loud enough to be heard: Now what do you think of your mindless, knife-happy surgeons? Dropped a note to Dr. Labmeister, too. And his boss; copy to Blazer.

Doctors can get their heads up their asses as far as anyone else. It's not that coordinating the care of GI bleeders had never been attempted, but turf issues and distrust had always prevailed. After a couple of particularly egregious episodes such as those above, it actually happened in my lifetime that we got a plan in place: massive bleeders went straight to the trauma service. People with less impressive bleeding went to the medical floor, but a surgical consult was mandatory for every one of them. It's incredible that such a thing had not been obvious forever. But Dr. Blaisdell was no politician: he had the unfortunate habit of speaking succinctly and plainly when he believed something. That he was right made it even worse. It had taken the arrival of a new chief of medicine, on whom Blazer hadn't yet trod, and to whom the rightness of the idea superseded any ego issues, to get agreement.

So partway into my stretch as senior trauma resident, timely consult requests for bleeding were no longer exceptional. Early in that new era, I was asked to see a young man, in his twenties. He'd vomited a couple of units of blood, then seemed to stop; about the time I saw him, he started again. He'd only needed about four pints, but the trend was clear. Surgery was not yet on the minds of his medical docs, but I convinced them that the time was right. After the operation—a very simple one-hour job I did with the help of the chief resident—I conspired to return the man to the medical ward whence he came, and handled his post-op care there. The medical folk got to witness something they'd not often seen: a simple recovery from an uncomplicated operation, a patient heading home happy and healthy. Reverse osmosis. Surgeons may have brass balls, but they don't have crystal ones. No one can say what would have happened had something been done differently. We make our best judgments, extrapolating from what we know. Picking the perfect time for intervention, choosing right every time is impossible. But I know this: with GI bleeders it's better to be a little early than to be too late. In that case, I'd say my timing was perfect.

The above-mentioned chief resident was Jim Holcroft—erudite and soft-spoken, both witty and serious, he's now a professor at the University of California, Davis, and among other things has carried on Dr. Blaisdell's interest in the physiology of shock. His academic leanings were evident early on. We had cared for a man brought in with severe hypothermia (low body temperature),

Cutting Remarks

who'd been found living under a bridge—drunk, disheveled, unconscious. Rewarming is fraught with peril; worse the longer the victim has been cold. As circulation returns, toxins from under-perfused tissues get washed back into the bloodstream; the liver and kidneys can fail, pancreatitis is common. The mortality rate is higher with each degree below normal. This poor man had been a popsicle, and he went through the whole menu of failing organs, dying after a couple of very miserable and complicated weeks. Jim presented the case at D and C conference in excruciating detail, relishing the physiological subtleties, oblivious to the shifting in their chairs and looking at their watches by everyone in the audience. After what I'd charitably call a thorough dissection of the case, Jim ended with the autopsy findings. The man, he said, had multiple hemorrhages in his gut. Dr. Dunphy was leading the conference, and Jim said to him, "This is very unusual. As you know, Dr. Dunphy, in the human the shock organ is the lung, whereas the gut is the shock organ in the canine." As Jim warmed to wrapping the whole thing up in a neat professorial package, and appeared ready to go for another half-hour, Dr. Dunphy interrupted. "Seems to me it's as simple as this: the man lived like a dog, and he died like a dog. Next case."

Holcroft was a terrific chief, and he taught me a lot, but my favorite recollection of him is mundane. On the trauma service, I lived on coffee and antacids. One morning on rounds, as Jim was talking, I reached into my pocket and popped a couple of Tums. Jim shot me a smile. "I like that," he said.

✳

Jesus returned to Earth while I was on the trauma team, and crash-landed. With shoulder-length brown hair, a manicured full beard, handsome, asthenic, and nearly naked, Jason Collins lay unconscious on the gurney, arms outstretched on arm-boards, Christ-like. Strapped to a hang-glider, he'd leapt from the cliffs near the VA hospital, got tangled, and shoveled into the beach. In addition to his head injury, he'd cracked several ribs, punctured both lungs, and appeared to have something bad going on in his belly. I liked to stand back and let the ER crew and the junior trauma team members do their thing, as long as it was going well. Several IVs, bilateral chest tubes, bladder catheter, X-rays. It gave me time to collect my thoughts, and in this case to wonder if Jason was as good a guy as he looked, and if so, whether he'd break the rule and live through this. (I've mentioned it: trauma survival being inversely related to societal value.) Severe head injury plus multiple other organ injuries means an uphill battle. Holcroft met me in the OR and I opened Jason up.

With trauma victims, we didn't dick around, always making a rapid incision from breast bone to pubic bone. It's about speed and exposure. Cut deep, top to bottom, through skin and fat, down to the muscle layer in one stroke. Then make a hole the rest of the way in, at the top. Insert your left index and middle finger, lift up and pull like hell. Poke the scalpel between the fingers with your right hand and, keeping the belly wall elevated to avoid cutting underlying organs, push both hands rapidly south, opening the belly like it had a zipper. When there's a lot of blood in there, you try to get it out as fast as possible to see what's broken. Scoop clots out with your hands; a suction device is too damn slow. Shove in huge cloth pads and haul them back out dripping blood, over and over; then pack fresh ones into the upper corners of the belly where the liver and spleen live. If the patient is unstable, you might use a big clamp to squeeze off the aorta, slowing blood flow into the belly. Take a quick inventory: any blood welling up from below? Toss the intestines from side to side to expose the retroperitoneum, looking for signs of injury. Once it's clear there aren't other things bleeding, you can head back to where the action is likely to be. Given blunt trauma and broken ribs, in this case that

The peritoneum is that shiny slippery layer that envelops the entire inner surface of the abdominal cavity, back and front. Behind it on the backside (the retroperitoneum) lie the kidneys, pancreas, aorta, vena cava and other assorted structures, injuries to which may present as retroperitoneal hematoma.

meant spleen and liver, both of which reside behind and are protected by the ribs. Jason had a small crack in his liver, which wasn't bleeding much, and which stopped with time and pressure. Good news. Major liver injuries can be enormously difficult to control. There was a small hematoma near the tail of his pancreas, and a shattered spleen, steadily leaking blood.

Most people get along fine without a spleen, which is fortunate because it's hard to put a fractured one back together. In those days, we rarely tried. The spleen does two things, mainly. It's a giant lymph node, so it has a role in fighting infections. But since the body is full of lymph nodes, immunity is rarely affected by

Not only is it often repaired currently, if a CAT scan shows a ruptured spleen with no other internal injuries, and the patient is stable, there might not even be an operation. It's especially worth the effort in kids, in whom the absence of a spleen can have greater immunity consequences than in an adult.

splenectomy; vaccinations help, too. And it's a filter: as blood cells age (their life expectancy is around 120 days) they get misshapen, and the spleen culls them from circulation. That function, too, can get handled elsewhere. So Jason got his spleen yanked out. Then a final pass around the abdomen, to be sure we hadn't missed anything. Spool the entire length of the bowel between the fingers, looking for tears. Check the hematoma to be sure it hadn't expanded. And close. Blazer insisted we use wire suture on all trauma cases. It made sense, in that wire is strong and non-reactive, meaning it would sit there and not become infected. But it was a pain, literally. Rather than tie it, we'd crank on it and twist, which left the edges of our palms below the pinkie fingers cracked, raw, and hurting. After a few twists, we'd snip with wire cutters, and turn the ends downward so they wouldn't poke the skin. Nevertheless, it often ended up uncomfortable for the patients. (One resident was sued for pain and suffering by a character who'd had them removed, several months after a spectacular save from a fatal barrage of gunfire issued by his fellow drug dealers.) I'll always consider Dr. Blaisdell a genius, but I never used wire after I left training, even for trauma. (As a matter of fact, Blazer himself published a paper a few years later, confirming the safety of using the newer forms of absorbable suture instead of wire. But I imagine he still insisted on neckties.)

Jason Collins had a complicated post-op course. He remained comatose, his punctured lungs kept leaking air, and he developed pancreatitis. His gorgeous girlfriend stayed with him the whole way, touching his unresponsive face and whispering to his unhearing ear. It was a tough go in the ICU, and it lasted a couple of weeks, after which he was transferred to the neuro ward, where he vegetated. I went there daily, checking on his chest tubes. As time passed, he aroused slightly; I'd find him in a chair, drooling into a plate of food, impassive, staring nowhere. At Amherst, there'd been a production of *Waiting for Godot,* in which the student who played Lucky stood hunched over and unmoving, mouth open, slobbering puddles onto the stage for an hour—a bravura performance if ever there was one. That's what Jason brought to mind, and it was a depressing sight. After a week or two, his lungs stopped leaking and I removed his tubes, making him a candidate for transfer to Laguna Honda Hospital, a dead-end for brain-damaged people. Saved from death, off he went.

It was nearly unheard of: a trauma patient returning to say thanks. Yet several months later, when I was chief resident, Jason appeared at the door to the ICU, accompanied by his girlfriend. The resurrection was complete: handsome and biblically hirsute as the day he'd arrived, he wanted to meet everyone who'd cared for him. He had no memory of his time there—none, in fact, of ever having been on a hang-glider. Other than that memory gap, and a few others randomly dispersed backward through his life, he was completely normal. That was a memorable day.

Faulty Volkswagen repair led to my biggest screwup as senior trauma resident. David Russell had an old Beetle, which he'd taken to have the brakes redone. He must not have checked out the work, because when he came to his first San Francisco hill and stepped on the pedal, it went all the way to the floor. Bracing his feet against the floorboard, he plowed into a tree at the bottom of the hill, his lap belt keeping him from going through the window. When they brought him in, he was in great pain, having broken both of his heels. He had a bruise on his belly from the belt but was otherwise stable. Prodding his abdomen and finding minimal pain, I decided his slight tenderness was consistent with the bruise. Belly X-rays didn't show anything amiss. (Plain X-rays of the belly are of limited value in evaluating trauma. If there's a major bowel injury, you might see air that's outside the bowel. CAT scans, as I've said, give an excellent look but weren't good enough or generally available then.) Having already admitted several patients to my overworked junior staff, I decided to let Mr. Russell go to the orthopedics floor and keep an eye on him myself. Deep in my brain, an alarm bell was ringing, but I managed to ignore it; we had more than enough to do that night. When I made it to ortho a couple of hours later, David's belly was a bit more tender, but his vital signs remained in the normal range, and I again managed to convince myself that everything was ok. There were a couple of other operations to do, so by the time I checked in again, another six hours had passed. Now his belly was tender all over, and rigid, impossible to ignore. (A rigid abdomen is a *sine qua non* of serious happenings inside: the abdominal muscles involuntarily tighten up, presumably to protect the insides from further injury.) With Holcroft doing another big case, the attending came in to help me do this one, and I was glad to have the chance to correct my error.

When I made the incision, I expected to see fluid or blood everywhere and was surprised to see the belly was dry. Had I been wrong about being wrong? Then I exposed the bile-stained and bubbly retroperitoneum on the right side, going all the way up and down David Russell's flank.

If you were to stomp on a very long water balloon, it would likely pooch out somewhere but not pop. If, however, you first closed off a segment with ties and stepped between them, it would have a good chance of bursting. That's why the duodenum gets blown out in certain seat belt injuries: it's the first part of the small intestine after the stomach, partly closed at the top by the outlet muscle of the stomach, and tethered for a long distance as it crosses to the left below the pancreas, behind the posterior peritoneum. The rest of the small intestine slithers around freely, and unless there are adhesions here and there it's much less likely to rupture from blunt force. Shoulder harnesses have improved things a lot, by distributing force across a broader zone. They weren't common then.

Timing has a lot to do with how you handle intestinal injuries, particularly colon and duodenum. The longer they simmer and seep before repair, the more contamination there is, and the more problems there are with sewing it up. By delaying Mr. Russell's operation, I'd blown any chance of simple and safe closure of the hole, and the defiled, dirty mess seemed to be shouting up at me, "You're a screwup and a lousy surgeon." I was sure the nurses and attending could hear it, too. An operating room has no hiding places.

One choice is to close the hole and leave plenty of drains in place; in other parts of the bowel a little leakage has a reasonable chance of drying up and healing on its own (assuming there's a route by which it can escape the abdomen—usually a drain tube of some sort). But this part of the duodenum is less likely to do so; it receives all the stomach content and bile in a straight shot, plus its blood supply is less rich than that of the downstream bowel. A leak can lead to a horrendous unending problem, and the time I'd lost meant simple closure was a huge gamble. So we did a "duodenal exclusion," which is a big deal: unhook the duodenum from the stomach (so food won't be passing by the hole) and close it off, while removing and closing off the bottom end of the stomach. Then you attach the small intestine to the stomach, just beyond the duodenum. It's a pretty neat bit of surgery, and I kept expecting Frank (the same Frank, by now an attending) to take it over.

How, after all, did I deserve doing a great case necessitated by my own mistake? But he let me keep going.

At the next D and C conference, the event was presented as delay in diagnosis: that Mr. Russell recovered didn't exculpate my original oversight. The main surgical point hammered in was that it takes a hell of a lot of force to break both heels; that kind of force transmitted through a lap belt is exactly what leads to duodenal injuries. To me the heels had been an excuse to finesse the patient to ortho, to give myself, and my interns, a break. That was the bigger message as far as I was concerned: you can't wish something away just because you're tired or busy. I've never seen another pair of broken heels, but I've been tired and busy a lot.

People who jumped off the Golden Gate Bridge never made it to the hospital, except for the rare soul who missed the water and hit dry land. Some of those—the ones that jumped near the end of the bridge—I think were aiming for salvation, and we were sometimes able to fix them up. I only saw one person who chose the Bay Bridge; he was pulled instantly out of the water by a providentially passing Coast Guard vessel and brought in still briefly semi-conscious. Not a mark on him, but his belly was expanding so rapidly and his pressure dropping so precipitously that I opened his chest and clamped his aorta there in the ER. (I've explained the value of clamping the aorta. Doing it in the chest avoids spilling blood until you're in the OR and half-way prepared.) This was one to pass up to the chief and the attending; I stood by as the abdomen was opened. When the blood was cleared away, his liver was floating unattached in the middle of his belly, torn completely away from the vena cava. Such is the power of rapid deceleration. Nothing to do but let the intern close the wound and call the coroner. I guess the man was serious, but the fact that he'd been alive and I'd talked to him before he passed out made me think he'd have liked, at that point, to have been rescued.

I still hate liver injuries. There's rarely middle ground: either they amount to very little, or they tax you to the end of your wits. It's the biggest organ in there, and its bulk impedes access to the very things that need attention, namely the veins connecting it to the vena cava. The blood doesn't even have the decency to spurt. It just wells up and continues like an overflowing sink, with no way to shut it off. All sorts of exotic maneuvers can be tried, including the Schrock shunt, invented by Ted Schrock while he was doing his lab year of residency right there. (More about him later.) It requires splitting the sternum, opening up a chamber of the heart, and threading a big tube down into the vena cava, beyond the liver, letting blood back to the heart without pouring out the liver. It works. Occasionally. Unless you and the patient are very lucky, you are bound to need uncountable pints of blood, to witness the loss of all clotting ability, and very possibly to end in defeat. It's hard to face a major liver injury without dread and pessimism. It's taken a return to ancient basics, in recent years, to improve the odds: stuff as many packs as you can in there, truss the liver like a turkey, and get the hell out. Come back another day to remove the packs, bit by bit. It works. Frequently.

seventeen

Able to Teach

"See one, do one, teach one" is the (mostly) ironic description of surgical training, as explained by surgeons. The numbers are wrong, but the concept applies. After an ill-defined period of looking and listening, you are allowed to hold the knife for longer and longer parts of an operation. Eventually you are talked and led through operations from start to finish, and it's assumed at some point you can figure out what you are doing. And if you know what you are doing, you ought to be able to show someone else. In the roughest of approximations, the intern is "see," the junior resident is "do," and the senior resident is "teach." (Of course, there's learning all along the way, nor does it stop at the end of training.) The obvious flaw is that the quality of the learning depends entirely on the quality of the teaching—more so in the absense of specified curricula. I've run into surgeons who seemed quite poorly prepared as they entered practice (especially those of more recent vintage), and others who were supremely capable. I think I was fortunate to have trained at UCSF, in that I learned a good way to handle most everything. Yet there was very little about my conduct of an operation twenty years later that was like that of my training. Narrowly constrained by the party line while in San Francisco, in my practice I was free to

Cutting Remarks

sample from my peers, from meetings and journals, and from my own ability to innovate. Which is exactly how it should be and, I'm certain, how it was intended.

If you were to ask nurses I've worked with after training, I doubt they'd say I'm either patient or tolerant of errors—especially my own. But as senior resident I surprised myself on several levels. I had a few things to teach and was an ok teacher. I found I could take a junior resident through an operation in a mutually satisfying way. Although you can't teach what you don't know, the process is at least as much one of learning as it is of showing. Assuming you know what the next step in an operation is, you can—as a teacher-assistant—make it pretty obvious by how you expose and stretch out an area of anatomy. Doing so not only leads the novice operator in the right direction, it reinforces what you know and allows you to discover new things along the way. There's an expectation as a junior doing an operation that the person on the other side of the table will show you where to go, or at least keep you from wandering too far off the path. When you're the teacher, you carry the weight on both sides of the table, and it has a way of crystallizing thought and focusing vision. It also makes clear how much was being done for you by your teachers in preceding years.

One of the first times I helped a junior resident take out a gallbladder, it turned out to be unexpectedly inflamed: thick, red, swollen, and stuck both to the liver and to the colon, obscuring the anatomy beyond easy recognition, creating a minefield. Make a step in the wrong direction to the north, get major liver hemorrhage; south, a hole in the colon; make a blunder to the east and you injure the main bile duct or the blood supply to the liver. (The ocean, as we know, is to the west, but you can't run out of the OR and take a swim, which is one of several ways by which surgical problems differ from medical ones.) I'd taken out a few severely inflamed gallbladders, but it was suddenly evident how much I'd relied on the more experienced assistant to establish planes for dissection. Showing good judgment or bad backbone, I called the attending in. And for the first time really saw how it's done. There are times for delicacy in surgery, and for brutality. Or a combination of both.

You can take a gallbladder out from the top down, or from the bottom up. Dealer's choice when it's healthy. When it's really inflamed, it's usually safer to start at the top, away from the bile duct, portal vein, hepatic arteries. No place for fancy dissecting scissors, no safety in smoking your way through with hot cautery, you work your way into the swollen tissues over the dome of the gallbladder. The tip of a suction catheter is a multi-purpose tool: you can insinuate it bit by bit, separating planes and keeping them vacuumed and visible as you go. When there's enough room, you can wiggle a finger in there. Pinching inflamed tissues between thumb and finger has a remarkable way of squeezing apart the abnormal and revealing the underlying anatomy. It's unlikely you'll pinch through something that ought to stay. And you can slide the tip of a right-angled clamp into an undecipherable layer and—the Dunphy rule—if you can see the jaws of the clamp through the tissue, it's safe to cut between them. Pretty soon you've got most of the gallbladder in the palm of your left hand, and you're safely working your way to the ducts and arteries. The same techniques work anywhere; an educated sucker, a well-chosen pinch, and a carefully placed angled clamp can bring order to all sorts of chaos. Delicate brutality. I learned it. There were times, in my practice, when I felt such a sense of triumph after a particularly tough dissection that I wanted to spike the organ on the operating room floor, like a running-back in the end zone. I pantomimed it a couple of times but always stopped short, figuring a splat wouldn't have the same dramatic effect as bouncing a football ten feet in the air. There was, however, the occasional fist-pumping "Yessss!!" along with passionate, if clumsy, dance moves.

When I found the courage to make a junior resident tear down a bowel anastomosis and do it over, I figured I was getting somewhere as a learner and a teacher. Bill Schecter had interned at the County and then left to do an anesthesia residency; when he returned as a junior surgery resident, he was a little rusty. I helped him do a colostomy takedown. (We did a lot of colostomies back then, as a way of dealing with colon injuries. After a time for healing, we'd hook the colons back up, and I'd done many such operations.) When he was finished, it didn't look right; a little mucosa was showing. Imperfect anastomoses leak, which is an unpleasant thing for all concerned. After the re-do, which looked a heck of a lot nicer, the patient did fine, and I took pleasure in the recognition that I was developing judgment. On another occasion, when Bill did an emergency tracheotomy with no time for supervision, I was the one to explain it to the attending. Bill has since told me he felt my support had a role in his being able to advance to the next year, knowing that latecomers didn't always make the cut. If true, it makes me proud: Bill is now Chief of Surgery at the County—brilliant, hard-working beyond the call, and a gentleman. Later, I'll tell you how he showed his gratitude by attacking me with a knife.

Judy and I had interns and junior residents over for dinner as often as possible. I considered them friends. It's hard to visualize them looking up to me in the way I did my seniors; I wonder if they did. The group was a different bunch from mine: there were artists, musicians, sportsmen. People who actually had and wanted a life beyond surgery. I had long talks with several of them, late at night in the call room, listening as they questioned whether this is what they ought to be doing. Some of their wives arranged a meeting with Dr. Dunphy to protest the long hours. Word had it he was more mystified than angry. The irony is that whereas a couple of them did drop out, most of them ended up like all the other UCSF trainees: a world-famous cancer surgeon, a chief of cardiac surgery at a big university, professors of surgery all across the country, busy private practitioners. I guess it's the obverse of the Trunkey rule: you can't unshine a surgeon.

One night I was having a particularly heart-felt conversation with an intern, standing by a window in a hallway. A body plummeted past the window, thumping onto a roof below. Unseeing, his back to the window, the intern talked on. I hated to interrupt, and I waited till the ER called before running down there. It was a prisoner, guarded in a private room, who'd managed to climb out a bathroom window. He ended up back in the same room, both arms in casts, legs in traction, finally shackled to his bed.

There had been times during my junior years when I, too, questioned the choice of surgery, one day in particular. Dozing on a rock above icy water near Dutch Flat, slowed down to a sleepy reverie by the hot sun, with Judy nearby (doggedly, you might say, avoiding the water), the realization penetrated my near-coma: this was the most relaxed and happy I'd been in months. It was a weekend off after a nearly non-stop couple of months in the hospital, made worse by a string of vacations by my counterparts. Is it ok, I wondered, to settle for a job you like less if it lets you enjoy your life more? That day it sure seemed so. Bill Hamilton, the head of the anesthesia department, loved to pick off surgical residents and seduce them into his program; it happened every couple of years, and he'd needle Dunphy triumphantly when it did. Anesthesia residents got the day off after they'd been up all night—how reasonable! I'd sidelonged an inquiry to Dr. Hamilton, who said he'd take me if I wanted to make the move. It's not that I didn't like surgery; it was just so, well, hard. Anesthesia wasn't exactly easy, but they seemed to have an enlightened set of priorities. On the other hand, they had to stand there and take crap from surgeons all day. My decision to stick it out was based on a guess: I looked across that swimming hole to the senior years and was pretty sure it would be better. It was. And that's what I told my interns and junior residents. Whether they believed it or not, they always went back to work.

To get the final patient of my senior year to the operating room, we had to call the Fire Department—for a second time. Julius Armstrong hadn't noticed the cops when he made the heist, and they were on his tail the minute he pulled away in his stolen Cadillac. They chased him at high speed toward Daly City, where he lost control in front of a junkyard, sliding sideways through a chain-link fence and stopping against a pile of pipe. If the doors of the Caddie were the lamb chunks on a shish-kebab, Julius was the red pepper: a two-inch diameter pipe had skewered the driver's door, both cheeks of Mr. Armstrong's buttocks, and the passenger door. Recognizing a low flight-risk if ever there was one, the cops waited for the Fire Department to arrive to cut him out of the car. They brought him into the Mission on a hand-held stretcher, which they had to tip sideways to get through the trauma room door—two or three feet of pipe sticking out crossways in each direction. Surgically, we were concerned about injury to his rectum, damage to the pelvic nerves, or tearing of major blood vessels, not bleeding now but ready to cut loose when the pipe was removed. With a hunk of metal obstructing the view, X-rays would be of no value. So he got the full trauma room production of IVs and catheters, prior to which we'd placed him on a gurney, and after which we realized we couldn't get him back out the door: he could no longer be tipped. Thus the call to the Fire Department to visit Julius Armstrong for a second time, for a closer trim. They arrived with sirens screaming, marched into the trauma room in full fire-combat gear, one of them brandishing a power saw. A couple of words of greeting, the whine of the blade, and the pipe ends fell away, the firemen exiting grinning.

After he went to sleep, we shaved and prepped Julius's abdomen for rapid entry to control blood vessels from inside, should it be necessary. It looked to me that the pipe was pretty loose, meaning it wasn't likely to be stopping any potential bleeding, but the attending was beside himself with anticipation of a heroic rescue. I scoped Julius's rectum; it looked intact, with no bleeding. We had a new medical student assigned to the service, and I let her do the honors: out came the pipe. Nothing. While the attending seemed to slump in disappointment, I probed around with my finger to be sure the sacrum felt ok, irrigated the wound copiously, placed a couple of drains, and that was it. Julius finished healing in the prison ward.

It's true more often than randomly: if you prepare for the worst, it seems less likely to happen. Get a urologist to run catheters backwards up the ureters when you think it might be hard to find them during a complex operation, and the ureters will be out of the way when you open. Don't do it, and it'll be impossible to find them. Have the nurses open a fancy and complicated set of retractors before you need them, and you never will. Crossmatch extra blood; the field will stay dry as goat's breath. (I have no experience with goat exhalations, but one of my future surgical partners loved that expression. I use it in remembrance of his premature death.) I doubt Mr. Armstrong would have bled to death before our eyes had we not been prepared, but it was a lesson that stuck.

Here's how things work in private practice nowadays: it costs extra money to crossmatch blood, so there's pressure just to check patients' blood type and screen for antibodies before surgery, because it's cheaper for the hospital. But if you get into the soup, it can take an hour or more to get properly matched blood. The lab will tell you that it only takes twenty minutes—but it never does. Moreover, there are quality assurance committees that look at blood utilization: if you order crossmatches but end up not using the blood, that's a black mark. You'll get a letter put in your file. So what's a surgeon to do? Worry about cost-cutting, or about being prepared? Let me know when you figure it out.

eighteen

Trauma, Chiefly

Becoming chief resident was as easy as moving one door down. Lacking comforts in many areas, the County nevertheless had a pleasant little suite for trauma call, which consisted of an outer room containing a couple of beds and enough furniture to house the previously mentioned collection of rectal implements and a few books, and to allow for small gatherings. The senior residents used that space. For the chief, there was a smaller inner room, which had bare walls, a bed, a bookshelf, a bedside table, and its own bathroom. Spartan and penitential as that may seem, it amounted to luxury and was well-deserved, since as trauma chief I wouldn't be leaving the building for sixty straight days. Don Trunkey did cover for me for one night: Judy and I went to see Steve Martin at a joint called "The Holy City Zoo." Martin was just beginning to be known, was still doing his arrow-through-the-head stuff. It was great to see him in a small venue. Afterwards, just to say I did it, I went home and slept in my own bed for a couple of hours. But I went back to work in the dark, so I still hadn't seen the light of day.

Judy brought food over some nights; we'd eat alone or share it with the senior resident. Sometimes I never made it to the room for the meal, stuck in the OR all night. Center of an abnormal existence though it was, I liked that call room, aware that it had housed chief surgical residents for decades, among them some great names in American surgical history. Whether or not I was a proper heir, I felt a sense of being at home there, as much as I did at our house on Cole Street.

I'd finished my senior year on the Trauma Service and stayed on to become chief. It had been my preference to do trauma at the end of my chief year, to go out on the crest of a wave. After all, being chief resident on trauma was the epitome of training, the position which for years had seemed impossible. What followed trauma would be anticlimax. Which, to some extent, it was. But things worked out fine. I moved my stuff into the chief's room and worked on becoming a surgeon.

It was more than I expected, and less. Seamless and without fanfare, it had been a natural progression. I wore the same white coat, with the same UC shoulder patch; no one could mistake me for an attending. Herb Caen printed nothing. (In the earlier days of SFGH—so we were told in a memorable lecture one day, sitting in an ancient amphitheater/lecture hall/operating room—the appointment of a new chief resident was announced in the paper. He'd then hear from two people: the local whoremaster who promised rewards in return for certifying his girls clean; and distillers seeking prescriptions for medicinal alcohol.) But my name tag now bore the designation "Chief Resident," and it felt pretty damn good. When I met patients and talked to them about their illness, explaining what we planned to do, I assumed they felt I wasn't an impostor. It was with me that the senior residents checked their plans, to me that they looked for instructions. I could pick and choose whatever cases I wanted to do, could be the one to help an intern or resident do it, teach them technique. In the morning I heard the intern presentations of the patients in our care, asked questions, and decided what needed doing for the day. I oversaw the management of the sickest people in San Francisco, in the ICU. At times I floated up and looked down at myself in amazement—this is really me, I'm doing this. In turn, I was constantly coordinating with the attendings, with Dr. Blaisdell, being held to account, questioned, instructed. Not as an equal—not ever—but it was palpably different. There seemed to be acknowledgement that I was nearly a surgeon, that what remained was polishing; it was no longer necessary to harass and harangue. That's how I saw it. I don't know what the hell the attendings saw.

Ben Fowler was the trauma attending when I started as chief. Tall and balding, usually smiling, he was so low-key and affable that he seemed to have wandered into the wrong place: Oops, sorry, I was looking for the mens' room. He had a slow, low-pitched rumble of a laugh, which continued on the inhale. "Huh, huh, huh, eeeehh, huh, huh, huh, eeeehh." Whatever I wanted to do was ok with Ben.

It's not that Ben ever refused to come in at night, it was just hard as hell to wake him up. Once I called around two a.m. about a lady with a perforated colon and told him my plan: remove the damaged portion, make a decision after I was in there about anastomsis or colostomy. Routine stuff. Ben was barely breathing on the other end of the phone. When I was done he said, slowly, almost inaudibly, struggling to remain in this world, "Ok, uh, just, uh, just don't, uh, just don't remove the larynx." Ok, Ben. Good plan. He knew he was a problem sleeper, often having no recollection of our conversations. One morning when he showed up for rounds

I greeted him by saying, "I did what you said about that kid, Ben. I still don't think the leg needed removing, but I guess you know best." It took him a moment to get the joke, which he did in time to avoid a change of underwear. Huh, huh, huh, eeeehh. Most often, in the middle of the night, the gunshots, the stab wounds, the GI bleeders—the everyday collection—I'd check in (such as it was) and then help the senior resident or do it myself. Finding myself willing and able to do those things alone at the beginning of my chief year was bracing. When the shit was hitting the fan, a little extra effort would always get Ben to roust himself and come in. He was there for the worst case I ever had, one that makes me sad and wakes me up even today.

Rebecca Olson was in her forties, had a husband and two beautiful and loving daughters, about eighteen and twenty. She'd found a lump in her breast and had it removed at a hospital in the East Bay. It was a small lump, and the procedure probably could have been handled with a local anesthetic. But it was done under general anesthesia—whether it was her or her doctors' preference, I don't know—and they'd had trouble inserting her breathing tube. Next day she'd had a low-grade fever and her pulse was up. She was having difficulty swallowing. It took another day for her doctors to realize her esophagus had been perforated when the anesthetist poked his tube down the wrong hole. And when

When you intubate someone—put a breathing tube into the trachea—you insert a flat-bladed instrument into the back of the throat to lift the tongue up and out of the way. The trachea and esophagus are stacked on top of each other like a double-barreled shotgun, with the trachea to the front of the neck. Hidden by the back of the tongue, it's sometimes quite difficult to see the entry into the airway. Intubating the esophagus instead of the trachea is not entirely rare, but the error is easy to recognize, especially nowadays. What is very rare is putting the tube into the esophagus in such a way as to perforate it.

they did figure it out, they made a too-small incision in her neck and stuck in a too-small drain, put her on too-small doses of antibiotics, and watched her get sicker for another day. As chief resident on trauma, their call was referred to me and I accepted her in transfer.

The center zone of your chest is called the mediastinum (mee-dee-uh-STY-num). It's the part that contains the esophagus, the trachea and its first branches toward the lungs, the heart, the thymus, the vagus nerves, a couple of other things. It's a tightly wrapped package, covered with a thin but tough membrane called the pleura, the chest's equivalent of the peritoneum. Once it gets a foothold, infection in the mediastinum—mediastinitis—is disproportionately virulent and hard to treat. Mrs. Olson's perforation had been undertreated long enough to have given the infection a major head start. She looked terrible: flushed, anxious, pulse thready and too fast, fever around 104. On her X-ray we saw widening of the upper mediastinum, with blurring of the edges, some air bubbles, and fluid around her lungs—all bad. I needed Ben's advice and presence for this one. We started big-gun antibiotics, opened her neck widely, gaining access deep into her mediastinum, placed several suction drains, and put in chest tubes on both sides. Next day she was noticeably less toxic. A swallow X-ray showed no sign of continued esophageal leak; maybe we could pull this one off. Scared and silent at the time of admission, her girls perked up and we had several conversations, increasingly cheerful.

When Rebecca's pulse and temperature went up a couple of days later, it was obvious that she was in trouble again. Now she had abscesses in her lungs. We opened her chest on both sides, explored her mediastinum from inside, placed more chest tubes and drains. Ben's unflappable attitude didn't reassure me. In fact, I wished he were as scared as I was. I bugged him two, three times a day: wasn't there something else to do? Having no prior experience with mediastinitis, I dug up articles, textbooks. I even went to Dr. Blaisdell. Just days ago a self-confident chief, now I felt impotent and brainless. Blazer was concerned enough to check with Dr. Fowler, but no changes came of it. Should we have done something differently at the beginning? Diverted her esophagus, opened her chest? Was Rebecca's fate sealed before we got to her? I was in her room all the time I wasn't operating on someone else. It went on for days. We operated again. If her daughters had me paged, I was there in an instant. Now she was on a ventilator, receiving medicines to strengthen her heart. She developed more and more abscesses in her lungs, too many and too small to drain. She swelled up, her former self washing away, helpless against the tide of her own fluids. Her kidneys started to fail. With infection rampant, she was moved to a separate room to the side of the ICU. Finally there were seizures, a sign of abscesses in her brain. A young woman, perfectly healthy a couple of weeks ago, not responding to any of our ministrations; her two daughters, towards whom I felt deep affection and painful sympathy, and with whom I'd talked for hours, sitting with her in tears as they realized she wasn't going to make it.

As Mrs. Olson's family said their goodbyes, I stood in the hall outside the room, choking up, hearing every word as I leaned against a window, hands on the sill to keep me from sliding to the floor. It had never felt right, it had seemed that we'd missed a chance. I didn't know then, and I still don't. Mr. Olson shook my hand, the daughters hugged and thanked me, said they knew I'd done everything I could; one of them kissed me. I never saw or heard from them again, except when I was named in the law-suit. I never learned how it turned out. Never tried.

At the D and C conference, Dr. Fowler took most of the questions. I was happy to stand silent. I can't remember what was said.

nineteen

Crumbs of the County

They tore San Francisco General Hospital down while I was there, hauled it away in a million buckets of murdered bricks. A new hospital was rising next to it, taking longer than expected, because the original was built tougher than anyone knew. Like some of its most notable patients, the County resisted its death to the end. I hated to see it go. Antiquated and inconvenient, it was nevertheless exactly what it should have been. Zen-like, it was the perfect embodiment of itself. The new building was, of course, more patient-friendly. It had private rooms, quiet and clean; but it was bland and blank. The open wards, the operating rooms with their tile galleries, seating an audience of all-but-visible surgical ghosts—gone. The connection to the history of medicine, real and unavoidable even to an exhausted resident, the sense that by entering that building you were stepping onto a path trod by pioneers: shattered by a wrecking ball, carted off without ceremony. Someone had, however, made off with a lot of money: the new walls were like those in a motor home. Open the doors too far, and they punched holes. Moving in was delayed because the elevator cars didn't fit the uneven shafts. Some equipment was broken or disappeared before it was ever used. But the transfer would happen during my tenure as trauma chief, and Dr. Blaisdell was adamant that the first operation in the new OR be done by the trauma team. The logistics were complex. For a while, we'd still be using the old Mish, and taking patients to the new OR.

It was a race with the orthopedists. Given Blazer's insistence, I was fully prepared to go out and stab someone myself, but the Tenderloin District produced when it counted, excreting a guy who'd been knifed in the neck. There was a fracture patient of some sort being teed up by the orthopods, so we rushed our neck wound to the OR before a thorough evaluation might show it wasn't needed. Nearly all penetrating neck wounds got explored: you've just seen the consequences of a missed injury to the esophagus. Vascular injuries could be subtle, too, blowing out after the fact. Years later, the use of various imaging techniques has allowed many necks safely to go unexplored. At the County, we erred on the side of having a look. In this case, it might have been a stretch. There was a little nick in the external jugular vein, no great threat, but it got us there. We won the race. As he did for all the chiefs, Dr. Blaisdell sent me a Trauma Team emblem and a congratulatory letter at the end of training. Mine included mention that I'd always be the first person to have operated in the new hospital. Hall of Fame stuff.

They saved part of the original structure, with its marble floor and curved wooden stairway, its elegant administrative offices. I don't know what came of the rectal repository: the call room went the way of the rest of the building. No one had considered the nightly needs of the residents. In the new hospital, we slept in what were to have been patient rooms—small and separate, empty of everything.

∗

Until they brought the victim in, I always thought those shotguns sticking up inside a police car were for crowd control. Scatter some little pellets their way, and people say, "Golly, I think I'll go home." The first barrel, in this case, had been used to gain entry through two inches of solid oak door; the next one emptied into our patient's right flank. The cops must have been fairly close, because the pattern of the pellets was tight. There were only a couple of exit wounds. The man was deceptively stable in the emergency room, before we took him upstairs.

Except in a food processor, I'd never seen liquefied liver before. I hope I never do again. In addition to the slurry in the right upper abdomen, the hepatic flexure of the colon was gone, leaving stool all over the place, and there were countless holes in the small intestine, leaking juices. I scooped away the hepato-fecal soup with my hands, uncovering a reasonable amount of intact liver, bleeding steadily but not beyond control. There was a huge raw surface, but the deep hepatic veins were intact. It looked like a salvageable injury. Placing several big sutures brought the bleeding down to an acceptable level, and I packed the area away to deal with the rest of the destruction. My attending was a surgeon from Northern California, participating in a visiting professor program Dr. Blaisdell had set up for his former trainees. Checking frequently to make sure the liver wasn't bleeding too much, we set about fixing the bowel injuries. There was no way to put the colon back together: it needed a double-barreled colostomy, bringing the ends on either side of the injury out to the skin. The small intestine had dozens of holes; so did the retroperitoneum over his right kidney, maybe his pancreas.

As we entered into the second or third hour of work, the patient began to ooze blood from everywhere; he'd received a few units

Cutting Remarks

of blood, but not enough to expect the sort of bleeding seen with massive transfusion. Was this Disseminated Intravascular Coagulation? If so, it would be desirable to get out of there as soon as possible, end the anesthetic, stabilize him in the ICU. Giving heparin (the blood-thinner showed by Blaisdell sometimes to work with DIC) won't solve the problem until you correct the underlying cause, and there were still countless holes in his bowel; you can't just leave them. We worked as fast as we could, but the bleeding got worse, now from the liver again, and from every injured area in his belly. Unavoidable, more blood was given, trying to keep the patient's volume up, but possibly compounding the bleeding problem. We always felt, on the trauma team, that if we could get a patient up to the OR, we'd get him back out alive. Not this time.

It's one thing to lose a patient when it's obvious there's an irreparable injury, like the man from the Bay Bridge. In this case, I'd thought we would save him; I'd gotten the liver under control, after all. No single one of his problems was fatal. Together, they added up to too much, but I wondered if anyone else could have saved him. When I presented the case at the D and C conference, I was alone, because the visiting attending had returned home. As I detailed the extent of his injuries and what we'd done, there was sympathetic nodding of heads in the audience, and no questions were asked. A barrelful of double-ought shot, at close range, is a lot of energy to absorb and walk away alive. Maybe I should have listed him as an error in diagnosis: he was dead on arrival, and we failed to recognize it.

Real men open chests in the emergency room. Every surgical resident wants to do it; it's exciting, dramatic, life-saving, and a little bit showy. We'd do it for any of several reasons, especially when there's massive bleeding in the belly: getting a clamp on the aorta via the chest can slow the leak of blood into the abdomen, without getting into a mess before you're in the operating room. Opening a belly in the emergency room for any reason—but especially for bleeding—would be disastrous. Because the belly wall compresses bleeding to some extent, pressure drops precipitously when you open and take away that compression, and you need all the resources of an OR to handle it.

More exciting, chests also get cracked for heart massage. When the heart is empty from exsanguination, pushing on the chest from the outside does no good, so we'd open chests directly to squeeze the heart until we could get the tank filled back up with blood and IV fluids. The desire to do it could be hard to resist. I stood watching, on one occasion, as the team was tuning up a victim of multiple gunshot wounds. He was semi-conscious, struggling and mumbling, fighting back reflexively at the efforts to help. Just after I turned away to call the OR and the attending, the patient hollered out in pain. Having heard the nurse announce the blood pressure had dropped to zero, the ER resident had started a slash in the chest.

"Holy shit!" I shouted as I turned back to the scene. "What are you doing?"

"Zero blood pressure. Gotta open the chest," he said, getting pumped up for the glory.

"Jesus Christ, man, the guy is awake!"

Reaching across the gurney, I fended off the attack before the scapel made it all the way in, leaving the resident to his own thoughts as we took the victim upstairs. No pulse, no blood pressure—the combination was often a ticket into the chest. But, c'mon, not in someone still talking and moving around! After a routine save in the operating room, stopping some bleeding, closing some holes, the man recovered without a problem. A couple of days after the surgery I casually asked him what he recalled about his time in the ER. Nothing.

There's a trick to emergency thoracotomy (opening the chest): ribs spread apart with difficulty, even in the OR. In an emergency, you cut between the ribs and toward the front, then turn the knife upward, making the shape of a hockey stick. To the side of the sternum, the ribs are all cartilage and cut easily. Slicing vertically through three or four cartilages makes an ugly scar, but it works: you can flip up the front of the chest like a trapdoor and get where you want to go. The most dramatic reason for thoracotomy in the ER, which we all wanted like a notch on a gun, is a stab wound to the heart (gunshots were rarely salvageable). It may not happen right away: a small stab allows blood to leak into the pericardium beat by beat, and as the pressure builds up it compresses the heart gradually (tamponade, as you've learned). Showing the typical sign of bulging neck veins as the blood backs up into the vena cava, the patient might fade away slowly. There could be time to get to the OR before opening the chest, maybe by sucking some blood out of the pericardium with a needle stuck in through the chest wall. With no time, you open in the ER.

If surgeons have a God-complex, this could be why: split open a chest, slice into the pericardium, stick your finger into a hole in the heart, and the patient may wake up with your hand buried in him half-way to the elbow. I did that once. The patient gave a thumbs-up to his friends as we wheeled him to the OR, the hole in his heart sucking on my finger like a hungry baby. At SFGH there were no cardiac surgeons, no pump techs. But it was self-selecting: a heart injury that might need bypass would have never made it to the OR. The ones that did could be fixed directly, by us. Holding the heart in your hand, compressing the hole with your thumb, enough also to dampen the beats as you place sutures on either side, timing your moves with the beating, aiming to avoid the coronary arteries—that's pretty cool. (Could it be cooler than scooping stool out of an abdomen?) When you place sutures into the heart muscle, it fires off a string of crazed beats, trying to jump out of your hand, not knowing you're there to help.

Victim of a drug deal gone bad, one fellow arrived in extremis and narrowly escaped ER thoracotomy. He'd been shot once in the lower abdomen and initially had barely measurable blood pressure, which was dropping steadily as his belly expanded. This was one of those ten-minute jobs, maybe faster. Several IVs, catheters in stomach and bladder, quick kidney check, ten units of blood sent to the OR ahead of us, and we were there. Splash iodine on his skin, be sure a couple of people were squeezing in blood, get the nod from anesthesia, open him up. As I did the "unzip" maneuver, blood gushed out of the belly. Bill Schecter, who was assisting, jabbed his hand into the wound to pinch off the aorta. Not a bad idea, if executed better. He hit my elbow, driving the scalpel into my left index finger, cutting to the bone. Bill pulled back as I said something terse. Controlling the aorta with my right hand, I held out my left to the nurse to see if she could tape up my finger. The digital artery was spurting enough that strips wouldn't stay put, and blood filled the finger of my glove every time I tried to put a new one on, bending back the flap of skin. We had already called Dr. Blaisdell, and when he arrived, I went to the ER to get sewn up.

By the time I made it back, Blazer was helping Bill repair a bullet wound in the left iliac artery, the main trunk to the leg. Damn. That was a good case. My case, thank you very much, Bill. (He says I remind him every time I see him. Surely I've forgotten it by now.)

The patient recovered without problems, so there was no reason to mention it at the D and C conference. When I finished my presentation for the week, Dr. Blaisdell spoke up. "Dr. Schwab seems to have forgotten the knife fight that broke out in the OR last week." He proceeded to recount the events of that night, getting a big kick out of it. Someone asked how the patient was doing, probably wondering if I'd poisoned him with my blood. "Doing fine," I said. "My blood brother. I expect him to be back out there selling drugs within a couple of weeks."

twenty

Whipple

When I finished trauma, my next rotation kept me at the County as chief on the Elective Service. ("Elective," by the way, means non-emergency: some people seem to think it means unnecessary.) Nice as it was to sleep in my own bed again, not alone, I missed trauma and was envious whenever I heard the team paged to the Mish. I know my writing hasn't done it justice: being chief resident on the trauma service at San Francisco General Hospital in 1976—there was nothing like it on the planet. There may have been other trauma centers as busy, but I'm pretty certain there were none in which you ate it, breathed it, slept it, infused yourself with trauma non-stop round the clock for sixty straight days. And it's not that learning trauma care *per se* was the point: to learn trauma surgery is to learn decision-making, rapidly assessing possibilities, considering options. It's gaining experience, over and over, with every technique a surgeon needs no matter the problem being faced, in the operating room and out. If you can handle being chief trauma resident at the County, you can handle anything. I'd done it. I'd become the guy I stared at as an intern, sitting in the D and C conferences, thinking it all but impossible. I felt if I were to leave and start a practice, I'd be ok. It might have been true. It also might have been the endorphin high of crossing the finish line of a marathon. I learned a heck of a lot more in the rest of my time there; and I still hadn't done a Whipple.

Deadliest of them all, cancer of the pancreas can only be cured if it turns you yellow the moment it arrives. Even then, the odds are grim. The dual-purpose pancreas lies crossways in the backside of your upper abdomen, in the retroperitoneum behind the stomach and duodenum, dribbling digestive enzymes into a duct running through its middle, and squirting insulin directly into the bloodstream. Through the part of the gland called the head passes the main bile duct, which joins with the pancreatic duct to empty bile and pancreatic juice into the first part of the duodenum, just past the end of the stomach. Behind it flows all the blood going from gut to liver, in the portal vein, and there are lots of little veins connecting from it to the backside of the pancreas. If a cancer starts right where the bile duct is, it may obstruct flow and cause jaundice (yellow color from bile in the blood). If it's small and early enough when that happens, you have a chance: you'll look funny before anything else happens, and someone will tell you to see a doctor. Any other starting point, it will have spread fatally before you even know it's there.

That's a lot of anatomy. Taking out the head of the pancreas and re-plumbing the area is a surgical *tour de force*, a blue-plate special that every surgical resident wants to sample. The operation is called pancreaticoduodenectomy, or the Whipple procedure, after the surgeon who invented it. Guy named Whipple. It requires removing the bottom end of the stomach, the gallbladder, the far end of the bile duct, the head of the pancreas, and the duodenum, peeling everything off the portal vein, sealing the branches, then reestablishing connections to the intestinal tract: anastomosing bile duct, pancreatic duct, and stomach sequentially to the small intestine. And if you're smart, you'll also put a feeding tube into the intestine somewhere downstream; if there are any leaks, the patient might not be eating for a while, and food into the gut works better than in an IV.

Painless jaundice and a gallbladder swollen enough to feel on exam—that's what Doris Wallace had when I saw her in the clinic, and those are the hallmarks of pancreatic cancer. (Among the other causes of jaundice, hepatitis doesn't cause a swollen gall-bladder, and obstructing gallstones aren't painless.) Tests showed something in the head of the pancreas, and no gallstones.

There are times when I've thought that having been inside people's bellies, touching them more intimately than they've ever been touched, knowing things about them that they'll never know themselves—seeing their *liver* ferchrissakes!—I ought to stay at their bedside for every minute of every day they remain the hospital. Maybe take them home with me. It's amazing still that people make the leap of faith required to let me operate on them. Not just me—it happens thousands of times a day all over the world. Whatever you might have heard about a surgeon, it can never be enough to make a fully factual decision. People need that faith. It's an honor to be chosen—surely it's that—and a responsibility which, if thoroughly considered, ought to be para-lyzing. But it's also less: if you're falling, you're going to hang onto anything (or anyone) within your grasp. Trust is not given; it's taken. A Whipple procedure was the biggest thing I'd ever proposed to do to someone whose life was not bleeding away in front of me. Mrs. Wallace said simply, "You're the doctor."

Blazer helped me, and it went fine. As opposed to the more typical residency time of eight or ten hours, it took us five. (Good, but still nearly twice as long as it would take me later in life—

and not good enough to keep Dr. Blaisdell from calling me "ham-bone" during the whole case. I'm pretty sure he called everyone that, in the OR.) Sewing bile duct to intestine is challenging in a fun way; they are of such different size and texture, the bowel with its inner layer trying to extrude out through the hole you make, that it's like attaching a giant noodle to a sweater and undershirt at the same time. The biggest deal is reattaching the pancreatic duct: digestive enzymes can digest anastomoses. When there are many ways to handle a problem, it usually means none is perfect. There are many ways to handle the pancreas in a Whipple procedure. Our choice worked out ok that day.

Because I wasn't brave enough to give her food, putting stress on all those anastomoses, I kept Mrs. Wallace on tube feeding for several days. It's a big incision; it took her a while to be up and around easily. Seeing her walking down the hall, I thought of all the work I'd done inside her, now invisible. She smiled at me, having no idea. How can such a thing ever make any sense? I'm no more than another human being. How could you let me do that? How could I choose to? I'd done big operations before. This one, for some reason, was different. Her simple acceptance in the face of such complexity embodied for me the mystery of surgery, the singular and honorable strangeness of the relationship between surgeon and patient, embedding it in me into a place from which it never left. Doris Wallace went home in a couple of weeks, recovering well, and came to clinic only once while I was on service. I never was back at the County after that, and lost track. She got a longer life from the operation. How much longer, I don't know.

✳

It annoyed Dr. Wylie that elective vascular surgery was allowed at the County, and at D and C conferences he'd leap on every complication that was announced from there. Trunkey helped me do a couple of big vascular operations, and we made sure not to give Wylie any meat. One was an aorto-bifemoral bypass—the Chevrolet of vascular procedures, involving taking a dacron tube shaped like an upside-down Y and attaching the one end to the aorta, the two to each of the main trunks to the legs, bypassing blockages. The other was a carotid endarterectomy—opening and cleaning out the main artery to the brain to prevent a big stroke or treat smaller ones. Vascular surgery is intense, and has a satisfying logic to it. It's also a battle you know you will eventually lose; blood vessel disease can be shoved back out the door, but it camps on your porch and always finds a way back in. General surgeons had always been the ones to do vascular surgery, but there was a shift underway to make it a separate specialty, requiring training after surgical residency. It made sense. I wasn't interested.

The Elective Service allowed equilibration, settling down from the consumptive demands of trauma into a life more like that of a practicing surgeon. I was doing a variety of operations at a manageable pace, in twelve- or fourteen-hour days that left time to spend with Judy and enjoy being in San Francisco, feeling like natives: Sunday morning coffee on our deck in the sun, becoming regulars at a few restaurants, having some time for friends and family. In the operating room, I enjoyed assisting and teaching junior residents as much as I did doing my own cases, learning as much from each. I worked with some new attendings: Bob Lim, expert in liver surgery, among many other things; Muriel Steele, who shared knowledge of colorectal disease; and Blaisdell, always Blaisdell. If it wasn't the adrenalin-infused, limit-testing, danger-producing existence of trauma, still the elective service was consolidating, allowing the coming together of who I was and what I wanted to be.

And then I left the County. After all those years, more hours by far than in any other place . . . the blood, toil, tears, and pus . . . growing up from watching lives being saved to actually doing it, myself, in the middle of endless nights. The place to which I gave everything, and which gave back in kind. Isn't that what love is? I walked out on a Monday morning, turned to look at the fading brick remnant and the high-rise engulfing it, and moved on, more sad than relieved, more perplexed than triumphant. There was no acknowledgement, not even a handshake. It felt like I was tip-toeing out on a lover, leaving a note on the pillow: call me.

twenty

Golden Colons

one

In one of the great disappointments of my training, Dr. Dunphy retired before I got back to the UC Hospital Gold Service (Dunphy's personal domain) as chief resident. Gold, as you've heard, was a mixture of staff and private patients—particularly, at that point, those of Ted Schrock, who'd been a chief resident when I was an intern and now was on the faculty. Nowhere near as outgoing and droll as Dunphy, Ted was an excellent operator—the best, I'd say, on the UC staff—and a committed, if occasionally dour, teacher. Because of his interest in inflammatory diseases of the bowel, there were lots of operations on people with Crohn's disease and ulcerative colitis—both of which can challenge all of a surgeon's technical skill and judgment. Not to mention those of the internists.

There weren't many GI bleeders at the UC hospital, so inflammatory bowel disease served as the stress point between medicine and surgery. Not long after arrival on Gold, I was asked to see a young man on the medical floor, admitted a couple of weeks earlier with an acute flare-up of ulcerative colitis. A process in which the inner lining of the colon becomes eroded, there's a broad spectrum of severity in which that disease presents itself.

Ulcerated areas may involve only a portion of the colon and respond fairly easily to treatment, or they can take over the entire length, bleeding massively and breaking down the barriers to infection. Surgery cures the disease, but often at a high price: the patient may have a permanent ileostomy, requiring a lifetime of wearing a bag to catch intestinal output. Lesser amounts of colon can sometimes be removed, hooking back up and avoiding the ostomy, but that leaves the door open for recurrent disease. Often successful, medical treatment—particularly back then—consists mainly of giving steroids. If surgeons are capable of giving ever higher doses of steroids to transplant patients, you can imagine what internists can do for inflamed bowels.

Being only twenty-three years old, the last thing Alan Miller wanted was an ileostomy. When he was admitted to the medical service, he'd been painfully passing clots of blood, and his colon, weakened by the disease, was stretching to a greater diameter than normal. But surgery was not on his mind, nor was it on the minds of his doctors. This was not a new diagnosis for Alan. He'd been on moderate-dose steroids for some time and had a mild case of the body changes that go along with it—rounded face, pot belly, thinned skin. Now he'd been getting increasingly higher doses of

An interesting issue: given the possibility of living with an ileostomy, there's some advantage to waiting until a patient is pretty sick with colitis before operating. It's amazing how much better people feel when ten pounds of chronically inflamed and infected colon is removed. For them, the trade-off is clear; many is the patient who has told me, after a few weeks of recovery, that they hadn't felt so well in years. Picking the right time— waiting long enough that they're ready, but not enough to get into trouble—is key. Another crystal ball thing.

intravenous drug, which had slowed but not stopped the bleeding, and which was accompanied by more dilatation of his colon.

That condition—megacolon, and its deadly sequel, toxic mega-colon, in which infection is passing through the colonic wall into the bloodstream—is a fearful complication, much to be avoided. Even in the most collegial and collaborative environments, decisions about managing inflammatory bowel disease are among the most difficult we make. How much drug is too much; when is surgical intervention called for; which operation, with or without making a stoma. Significant adverse consequences are possible with any treatment. When I saw Alan Miller, he was way beyond the head-scratching phase. His colon was of a size where perforation was imminent, and he was still bleeding; the time for a consult had long since passed. Once again, in the training-program tug-of-war between surgeon and internist, the patient was the loser. Alan was sick, ready to sign up for anything that might make him feel better, but he was now on massive doses of steroids, making healing questionable, and post-op infection a near-certainty. Ted Schrock had no hesitation in agreeing with me; in fact, he was initially angry, assuming that I had surely been consulted earlier and had allowed Alan to get to this point.

Desperate to save itself, the body has the ability to plug holes in the bowel. Hanging down from the transverse colon like an apron, the omentum is a thin, roughly square sheet of fat imaginatively referred to as the policeman of the abdomen. Where there's trouble, there it is: floating around in front of the intestines, it will stick to an area of inflammation, and in doing so it both prevents or seals leaks, and provides an extra conduit for healing cells to find their way into the war zone. The small intestines can stick and

It's noteworthy that a majority of colloquial medical descriptions involve food: nutmeg liver, chocolate cysts, cherry angioma. Perhaps in calling the omentum a policeman, the reference was to doughnuts.

form a local barricade as well. Those processes can save a life, but it can create a hell of a mess for a surgeon.

Alan Miller's colon, it turns out, had perforated in several places. Preventing the outflow of stool, the omentum and small bowel were adherent to it at each hole, denoting a situation much worse than had been clinically apparent. (That's another danger of high-dose steroids: they not only reduce immunity but suppress some of the usual responses to infection, such as fever. A patient can look and even feel well while disaster percolates inside.) To get Alan's colon out, I had to unravel and cut through knot after knot of twisted bowel and omentum, unroofing several contained abscesses, trying not to create holes in his small bowel, made thin and fragile by the steroids. Tough stuff. Ted was at his best in those situations. I learned from him more than anyone else how to manage difficult dissections of bowel. Our only choice was to remove the entire colon and give him an ileostomy (bringing the end of the small intestine to the skin).

Had he been much older, or had he had other medical problems, I doubt Alan Miller would have made it. His ileostomy wouldn't heal to the skin and lay in a puddle of soupy tissue, leaking around the bag. His main incision fell apart, despite using monster reinforcing sutures and leaving the skin open to avoid trapping infection underneath. He developed fistulae in his small intestine, no doubt from areas we'd weakened in our dissection; usually, suturing such nicks prevents a problem. Not when there's infection all over; not in the face of the astronomical dose of steroids he'd gotten. Intestinal fistulae had been one of Dr. Dunphy's interests, and the Gold Service had plenty of experience with them. Before hyper-alimentation (high-calorie intravenous feedings), there was often no choice; you'd have to go back in and try to close the holes. But early in the healing process, tissues are so dense and uncompliant that it could be nearly impossible, and the dissection would create even more holes. Dunphy, and others, showed the value of waiting. First, many fistulae will heal on their own, if the output isn't too high and if there's no obstruction downstream. Second, after time, adhesions soften and even disappear, making reoperation immeasurably safer and easier. So we plugged Alan into an IV, fashioned some drainage devices to lay in his wound, and stood back. For two months.

Like that of the woman I'd seen on Gold years ago, Alan's wound contracted and healed over, covering everything except the fistula holes. His ileostomy solidified, and he gained weight and returned to reasonable health. Now on normal levels of steroids, when I reoperated to remove the section of fistulized bowel, re-do his ileostomy, and close his incisional hernia, he recovered easily and went home well, after more than three months in the hospital. Having had removed five feet of chronically sick and festering colon, with which he'd been living for years, he said he felt better than he'd thought possible. Since training, whenever I've been asked to see a patient with ulcerative colitis, Alan Miller taps me on the shoulder.

I saw many cases of Crohn's disease as well. Equally as mysterious (the cause of each is unknown), and more variegated than ulcerative colitis, Crohn's (also called regional enteritis) can affect any part of the intestinal tract, famously creating "skip areas" wherein diseased segments are scattered about with normal areas in between. Most often, it involves the very end of the small intestine (the terminal ileum), right where it joins the colon. A typical zone of regional enteritis causes the normally soft and snakey bowel to look and act like a blood sausage—inert and obstructive, causing pain, blockages, and the sort of unwellness you'd expect if you had a hunk of spoiled meat inside you. Unlike ulcerative colitis, Crohn's disease is not generally cured by surgery; recurrence happens at least half the time. But people sick enough with it can get enormous and usually long-lasting relief by having the segment removed. In nearly all cases, it's possible to reattach the ends of the removed section; patients are well and happy, without the need for a stoma. However, unlike taking out a colon—which doesn't affect digestion—removal of more than a small amount of ileum can cause nutritional deficits. So once again, selecting the perfect time for and extent of surgical intervention is a challenge to everyone involved. I'm happy to say I don't recall any disasters in that regard. My point in bringing up Crohn's disease is that seeing a lot of it helped to form judgment about operating. And more importantly, I gained experience in handling such abnormal bowel as is seen in the disease. Freeing it from its surrounds, deciding how much to remove, handling the distortions of tissue caused by chronic inflammation, making one anastomosis after another, managing post-op steroid doses—the Gold Service of Ted Schrock and his patients taught me a lot. Including seeing the rectum as more than an implement receptacle.

The colon's job is to absorb water: after digestion in the small intestine, the leftover undigestible stuff flows into the colon, passage through which changes the liquid into a manageable solid. Absence of colon means having less than solid bowel output, but no nutrients are lost (generally speaking).

The rectum, anatomically speaking, is that part of the colon which leaves the abdominal cavity and dives through the pelvis, fully surrounded by bone, on its way to the outside world. Especially in males, with their narrow passageway, that pelvic portion is a tough place in which to operate, the most challenging of any portion of the colon.

What you try to do is find the exact plane between the backside of the rectum and the sacral bone, and start there. If in the perfect place, wiggling your hand downward creates a sort of slurpy sucking sound as the tissues separate—hearing it is audible confirmation you're where you want to be. As things loosen up, bloodlessly, you can insinuate your fingers forward around one side of the rectum and then the other, eventually working your way to the front, cutting between your fingers with a cautery device on an extra-long handle. Because it's deep and narrow, and your hand obstructs view of what's beyond, it's done largely by feel. Getting beyond the tumor (which is the most frequent reason you'd be doing the operation) with enough room to cure it, and leaving enough rectum or anus to hook back up to—avoiding colostomy— is ideal, but it can tax both judgment and technical skill. (Here's an area where stapling devices have made a huge difference, allowing surgeons to avoid making colostomies in situations that previously required them.) I have pretty big hands ("How did you get that gallbladder out through such a tiny hole, with those hands?"), and folding them up to work in the pelvis often led to painful cramping: I'd have to stop and shake them out frequently, making me understand the surgeon who scared the father of my medical school roommate into becoming a psychiatrist. When he was a medical student, he developed an infection in the bone of the tip of his pinkie finger. The doctor who saw him offered to remove the entire finger, all the way through the palm, saying it would give him a great advantage if he chose to become a surgeon. There were times, cramping my way through a pelvic dissection, that I thought about it.

Most sinister of all pelvic hazards are the pre-sacral veins. Just off that perfect plane between sacrum and rectum, paper-thin and fragile, spread out and stuck to the bone like a starfish on a rock, runs a network of pelvic veins. If you get into them, the bleeding can be nearly impossible to stop because, due to the way they're attached to the bone, it's hard to get instruments around the veins without tearing them more. People have bled to death despite—or because of—surgeons' attempts at control. I watched it happen when I was an intern. I got into them once, several years later, in practice. Tipping the lady nearly onto her head to drain blood away from the area, I had the idea of cutting up pieces of absorbable cellulose cloth used to stop bleeding, loading them onto thumbtacks and pushing them into the sacrum through the veins. In a desperate situation, the nurses were willing to scrounge tacks from a desk somewhere, cook them up in the sterilizer, and hand them in. It worked perfectly, and I saw the lady for years afterward, cured of cancer and happy.

Some months later, another surgeon got into the same pickle. (Try not to worry: it's actually pretty rare.) As he was losing the battle, one of the nurses told him I'd done something to solve the problem. I wasn't around but Joanie was, and she went into the OR to talk them through it. It worked again. But that was enough to get word to higher places: never again, we were told, would the use of "non-surgical" thumbtacks be allowed in an operation. As far as I'm concerned, stainless steel is stainless steel: it's used all the time in operations. Hip joints are setting off airport alarms even as you read this. I couldn't see the problem. Rising to the occasion, a surgical supply company now makes thumbtacks, indistinguishable from the office variety, and charges, I have no doubt, a couple hundred bucks apiece.

Next to a Whipple, the biggest operation a surgical resident can do is esophagogastrectomy. Required for cancer of the distal esophagus, nearest to the junction with the stomach, it involves cutting loose from all attachments the entire stomach, until it's dangling between the esophagus and duodenum like a hammock. Having done that, you close up the belly, turn the patient on his side, and open the right chest (there are ways to make a single incision, but this is the best approach), pulling the stomach up into the chest. Then, the upper half of the stomach and the lower half of the esophagus are removed, taking the tumor along with them. Reattaching the esophagus to the stomach, deep in the chest, is among the more difficult and tenuous suturing jobs a general surgeon does. (It's another area, currently, where staplers have made a big difference.) Emblematic of the perverse side of that surgeon-patient relationship, I was glad when Mr. Holden showed up in clinic with esophageal cancer. I planned, I did it in my head, I re-read texts; so I was disappointed—for myself!—when we operated and found a single tiny deposit of cancer just outside the operative field. This was to have been my first, and I had to suppress the urge to say something in protest as Ted decided there was no point in proceeding; it wouldn't be curative. Instead, we placed an enormous tube in his esophagus, shaped like a funnel with an extended spout, traversing the tumor location and anchored to the inside of the stomach. Its purpose is to prevent obstruction, allowing at least the swallowing of saliva, if not food. In case he couldn't eat, we also placed a feeding tube into his stomach and closed up.

Mr. Holden stayed on our service as he recovered and began radiation treatments. Scholarly, with a tidy mustache and grey hair below his collar, he reminded me of a professor I'd had in college. We talked small, we talked literate, and I tried to be both upbeat and realistic with him. He wanted as much time as he could get, but one day he didn't return from radiation. The tube, the tumor, the radiation had all worked together to erode a hole into his aorta, and he died in an instant. He'd have been better off, I think, had we gone ahead with the operation. After that third case of erosion into a major artery, I've never seen one again.

twenty

Necks Case

two

Stones, bones, and groans. It's the mnemonic for the classic symptoms of hyperparathyroidism. Among the endocrine glands, the parathyroids are the most variable in number and location. Hiding behind the thyroid in the front part of neck (usually), they are four in number (usually), brownish in color, and about the size of a pea. They secrete a hormone that controls the level of calcium in the blood. The level of secretion is (usually) regulated by the pituitary gland, in the brain. Parathormone works by making the bones release calcium. If one or more parathyroid glands (usually only one) develops a tumor within it (usually benign), it can produce unrestrained amounts of parathormone, which causes abnormal entry of calcium into the blood, which can precipitate in the urine (stones), cause osteoporosis as it weakens the skeleton (bones), and deposit in the pancreas, causing pancreatitis (groans).

Before the days of automated screening blood tests, calcium levels were not routinely measured, and the condition was diagnosed far along the pathway to trouble. In the 1970s, such tests were becoming widespread and, to the surprise of many, it was discovered that lots of people walk around with elevated calcium levels and tumors in their parathyroids. The disease was being picked up before any symptoms. As uncommon as hyperparathyroidism had been as a surgical disease, it was now becoming commonplace (which suggests that many of those people would have been perfectly well-off had they never had a blood test). Between Maurice Galante and Lester Weisman on Blue, Tom Hunt on Gold, and Orlo Clark at the VA (I haven't mentioned him: another former resident now on staff who has become a world leader in endocrine surgery), necks were being plucked at UCSF like a backyard grape arbor.

I'd assisted Tom Hunt with several of his private patients on Gold. When a clinic patient with hyperparathyroidism came along, Tom told me to take care of it and call him if I needed help. Imaging studies have made the operation more predictable now, but then it was a matter of getting there and having a look, searching where the glands are most likely to be, and then—if they weren't there—in all the other possible places: behind the carotid, the esophagus, in the upper mediastinum, sometimes inside the thyroid. They've even been found in the abdomen.

There are operations that are physically exhausting, demanding brute effort paid for with sore back, aching neck, wobbly legs. There are operations that are mentally draining, requiring dangling right on the edge of disaster, focusing intently for hours on end, worrying about a wrong move. Parathyroidectomy is unique: it's easy to get there, and the work is pretty safe once you've arrived. It's just damnably, annoyingly, embarrassingly, flop-sweat-producingly frustrating. Or it's not. You can find the abnormal gland easily, looking like a genius, done in half an hour; or you can search and search, feeling the glare of everyone in the room, not wanting to catch their gaze, going back and back to the same places, looking again, working through the list of less and less likely possibilities, thinking it would feel less awkward if you'd wandered naked into a garden party. So after a couple of hours, I called Dr. Hunt. He walked in and looked over my shoulder, walked out and scrubbed, came back, asked for a forceps, and plucked the goddamn gland out in about two seconds. "See that artery?" he asked, pointing at a branch the size of a grain of rice (uncooked). "It's bigger than it ought to be. It's feeding the tumor." Oh well. I guess it's called experience. The case didn't deter me. I still liked working in the neck, and I eventually figured out how to find those things, pulling out plums of my own.

It hit me when I first operated on a patient with thyrotoxicosis—wherein the thyroid over-produces its metabolism-regulating hormone, heating a body like a boiler ready to blow. My biological father, the internist, had died post-operatively, having had his thyroid removed for that very condition. In the 1940s, the aptly named "thyroid storm" was a much-feared and often-seen complication. Surgical manipulation squeezed hormone into the bloodstream, anesthesia muted the body's protective responses, and within hours of surgery the pulse, blood pressure, temperature could go up and off-scale with deadly result. Because of more effective drugs with which to cool down the gland before operating, and which counter the stimulating effect of the thyroid hormone during surgery, thyroid storm was rare in the '70s and is about non-existent now. I'm no shrink. I'd given no thought to the factors that made me choose medicine, and then surgery, and then the kind that did thyroid operations, until I found myself doing the very operation that had killed my father, having made the simple preparations that would have saved him. As I entered the OR, I wondered: would it be a B-movie moment, a zoom-in on my sweaty brow as I froze up, the nurse looking worried, asking, "Is something wrong, doctor?" It didn't happen. The operation flowed like any other. Had it been a way of meeting the man I never knew, and who never knew me? Of symbolically saving his life, while the quest saved my own? A meeting of souls in the ether, as it were? I've thought about it a lot since then. I like the idea, but I'm pretty sure the answer is no.

Near the end of my time on Gold, I took a call from a nursing home. A long-time resident had developed fever and was draining fluid from her abdomen. In her seventies and looking much older, Mrs. Ross had been a life-long alcoholic who'd destroyed most of her pancreas over the years, along with much of her brain. We admitted her to a four-person room, where evaluation showed her to be marginally alert, unaware of who or where she was. Her chest X-ray indicated pneumonia, and her family, seeing a painless way out, requested that we attend only to comfort, and let her go. Across from her bed was a woman not much more awake, who—as was later pieced together—sometime in the night made a friendly offer of a cigarette to Mrs. Ross. On my arrival the next morning, the nurses described the sight of Mrs. Ross wandering out of her room, her gown in flames. Having already made the decision not to treat her pneumonia, it made sense not to become aggressive with burn treatment. Rather than transfer her to the burn unit at the County, we kept her and simply increased her pain meds. When she died, I wondered how to explain it at D and C conference. You've already read how I tried and failed to slip it by.

Which provides the opportunity to expand on that conference called "D and C." Most places call it "M and M," for Morbidity and

Mortality. The UCSF nomenclature, it seems to me, speaks a vivid truth: "D and C" as a term is better known as an abbreviation for Dilatation and Curettage—stretching open and scraping out the uterus. And that's exactly how it felt when Deaths and Complications were addressed. Rarely was a thing glossed over. Elevated stature among the faculty afforded no exemption, particularly because there were a few retired profs who'd show up and talk straight. I especially liked Brody Stephens, wiry and compact, maybe in his late seventies, who wore perfectly tailored three-piece suits with a flower in the lapel and called everyone "pal." He was still doing a bit of surgery when I started—thoracic mostly—and when he'd appear on the wards he'd be grinning with a nurse on his arm, well aware that the nurses considered him cute, working it. At one conference, Philip Griswold was being hammered over a bad outcome. He eventually gave up and said, "Well, I guess I might have done the wrong operation." Brody said, "You did the right operation, Phil. You just did it wrong." Or, if he sensed a bit of big-wigged fudging, he'd stand up and ask Dunphy: "What do you think, Bert? That's not right, is it? Tell us what you think, Bert."

What can you say about post-op bleeding? What was heard at D and C conferences, over and over, was this: "It was dry when we closed, Doctor Dunphy." So often, in fact, that one chief finally arrived at a laudable shorthand. Announcing a reoperation for bleeding, he took just the initials of that sentence and said, "I.W.D.W.W.C.,D.D." A moment's reflection, then a reverberating laugh from Dunphy, and no further questions. That trick got a lot of chiefs off the hook during the Dunphy years.

Dr. Dunphy had a thing about post-operative urinary retention (the inability to urinate after surgery, requiring insertion of a catheter). He felt it should never happen, and that when it did, it was an intern failure. We should run water, he said. We should do what he did when he was an intern: stand on a chair by the patient's bed, pouring a bucket of water into another bucket on the floor. We'd hear the lecture a few times a year. Otherwise, when the chief mentioned urinary retention, Dr. Dunphy would just smile and roll his eyes. I've always wondered how many patients were scared pissless by an intern, afraid of becoming a statistic, asking over and over, "Did you pee yet?" a bucket of water at the ready. (After Bert Dunphy retired and Paul Ebert took over, urinary retention was exempted from mention. In fact, the D and C conference seemed in general a lesser priority to Ebert. Too bad.)

Serious issues brought serious discussion, and that's where the learning occurred. Anastomotic leak: what prep had been done, should a drain have been placed, a stoma created? Wound dehiscence (incision falling apart, often with some amount of evisceration): what suture? How far apart? Too tight? Were retention sutures used (big extra buttressing stitches)? How was the skin managed? When deaths occurred, unless it was judged inevitable, every option was scraped out and examined: was the operation too soon, or too late? Should a different one have been done? Or none at all? Was it done properly? It could be brutal, and could go on for hours. Dr. Dunphy could cut to the bone and, when tension threatened to explode, he could cut that, as you've heard, with a perfectly timed wisecrack. And, if well-placed, he didn't mind the occasional one from a chief resident.

The Master's Voice

Omigod. After all these years, so close to the end, and I don't know a damn thing! In an endless soliloquy, Dr. Victor Richards is pointing out my inadequacies to everyone in the operating room. "Look at that. Look at that! Isn't that something? He doesn't see it! He had it, and he lost it. There it is! No, he lost it again. Slow down, Dockie, you're going too fast. I'm the slowest surgeon in town. Stop a minute, Dockie! Study it. Just look at it. See that? Look how it slides. Look at that! He's moving. He can't stay still. The great American urge to be on the move. He's hitting the packs. See that? He did it again. Steady it. Isn't that something? Isn't that something? Look at that! Stop. Put a little pressure on it. Since the days of Attila the Hun, they knew pressure stops bleeding. Wait. When there's nothing to do, do nothing."

In those years in the anatomy lab, and in his practice ever since, Vic had rewritten the rules, found his own way to make melody in the OR. And now, to my left, leaning, shouldering me like a power forward, reaching in front of me and poking around, he's trying to get me to hear his song, while drowning it out with frenetic, insistent, non-stop talk.

Back at Childrens' Hospital for the final months of my training (I'd had to choose between being chief with Vic, or at the VA
Hospital), I am finally where I thought I'd wanted to spend some
time, learning from the master. Now I'm not so sure. From the
most mundane to the most complex, there was nothing he did
that was the way I'd been taught. I'm on another planet,
unschooled in the language. And Vic, while anxious to teach, had
a hard time slowing his mind down to human speed. Knowing
there was information passing me by, trying to keep up was
exhausting and frustrating: I am drinking from Niagara Falls with
a paper cup.

I've already filled this book overmuch with surgical detail. It
would take volumes to make understandable the extent to which
Dr. Richards changed my approach to surgery. No concept
remained the same. He'd thought about everything, from the
simple to the most complex, using efficiency and his unique
knowledge of anatomy as the guiding principles. "Make the ends
even," he'd say as I placed a suture and made ready to tie. It's
easier—it should have been obvious—and saves a few seconds.
Packing away the bowel was an obsession: working in the belly,
you're displacing the intestines from where you are attending,
and they want back. Lots of surgeons roll up pads and stuff them
here and there, holding the guts away, and just accept that at
some point a loop will squirt its way back into the field and need
another wad of gauze. Not Vic. For every corner of the abdomen,
for whatever operation was being done, he'd found a way to
insert packs once, holding the field open for the duration. He'd
let me struggle then show me the way: put the corner here, fold
it like this, lay another on top, tuck it there. Each move made
sense; none needed repeating. Each instrument was the right

one, and if it could be made to serve multiple functions, eliminating the need to hand it off and get another, that's what would happen. Cut with a knife, spin it in your fingers, and use the handle to slide through a layer, turn it back and cut again. Resist the scrub nurse's insistence that you put down a dissecting scissor and use a different one to cut suture. It's amazing how much time is wasted in an operating room.

Most important, and most difficult to assimilate, is the concept of layers. "Study it, look at it a minute, see it slide." Adjacent structures are not glued together. There's a plane, delicate and exact, that separates them. Get in exactly the right place and you can move about easily, not leaving a footprint, not spilling blood. It's the difference between gliding on ice and walking in sand. So while dissecting, Vic would subtly move the tissues as he approached his target, producing the slightest slide between elements as the plane revealed itself. Then, a finger, the handle of a knife, the back of a scissor, flicked across the field, and the axillary vein, the external oblique fascia, the mesenteric artery, were laid out in an incomprehensible instant, glistening clean and ready to submit.

For every operation, Vic had an anatomical secret. Inguinal hernia, surgical bread and butter: slide a clamp along the "reflex inguinal ligament" (did he discover that? I'd never heard the term) and the awkward and gross struggle of encircling the spermatic cord (the structures going to the testicle, through which the majority of male groin hernias occur) becomes easy and gentle. Work a bit on the outside surface of the spleen, and you can deliver it into the incision ("the spleen is a midline structure, dockie"), making removal a twenty-minute breeze. He was the one who showed me how to pop a thyroid out of the neck. He made easy the often-difficult task of clearing fat off the surface of bowel, readying for anastomosis. (Who opened that window? It's not fat in here anymore.) Vic showed me that I'd been making appendectomy incisions in the wrong place, too much toward the middle, as I'd been taught. Make it more to the side, and the little worm is right there, no struggle, no rooting around. And so much more. We did every operation in general surgery, eighteen a week—gastrectomy, hernia, mastectomy, thyroidectomy, big cancers, little zits, on and on. A couple of esophagogastrectomies. Always with the patter, the cajoling.

"He's not seeing it! He had it, and he lost it." He was right: I didn't see it, for a discouragingly long time. Like every other surgeon, I could do those operations, making it happen in a satisfactory way, adequate, not knowing there was a more logical way, a faster way, a way of poetic beauty. I've already said it: it may not always make a difference to the patient—it usually doesn't—but it came to make a difference to me.

Eventually, I started to get it. Planes revealed themselves to my wiggling finger. In place of the harangue, there began to be words of approval. Seeds took root, although it took a couple more years to see the blooms. In practice, my surgical times were like Vic's (faster, since I didn't have me holding me back), as were my outcomes. (Fast, by the way, is neither a necessary nor sufficient characteristic of good surgery. But comparing two properly done operations, the quicker will see fewer post-op problems than the longer one, given enough instances, especially in sick people.) There have been times when I've let myself imagine Vic watching me operate, thinking he'd be proud, despite (or perhaps because of) the fact that there's very little I did later that was exactly the way Vic taught. Such times don't last: it's become clear to me over the years that there are special gods of surgery who scan the land looking for surgeons feeling good about themselves. Allowing no more than a couple of days of self-esteem, they fire off a bolt of reality, in the form of a complication, or a case that makes you feel like an incompetent slug.

In no way as brilliant as Vic, I shared some of his quirks and interests. I like making rounds in the most efficient route possible. I hate fussy bandages. I want each move to have a good reason—"that's the way I was taught" isn't among them. We talked politics, philosophy, music. I was interested in the lives of his patients. When such conversions took place in the OR, I took it as the ultimate sign of approval, the diatribe becoming less intense. He invited me to the Bohemian Club, an exclusive hoidy-toidy East Coast sort of place, peopled with the uber-rich and influential. I felt like a crumb on a tablecloth, but the food was good. And Vic took special pride in the fact that Judy got pregnant while I was on his service. Avoiding the gory details, we'd been through a not-atypical yuppie infertility thing, to the resolution of which the stresses of the UC experience were not especially conducive. ("Be back in thirteen minutes, boys. Judy's scheduled for an in-vivo semen analysis." Cole Street was about five minutes from Moffitt.) Vic thought a chief resident shouldn't have to kill himself: "Go home. Enjoy life." When Daniel was born, while we were living in Oregon, Vic sent him a silver baby cup.

Nearly as life-altering, I got one non-surgical gift from my time with Dr. Richards. I removed the gallbladder of the wife of a theater owner—the only one in San Francisco where *Star Wars* was playing. This was the first one, and lines were blocks long, people waiting hours to get in, private cops and portable toilets ensuring civility. A lover of science fiction, I longed to see the movie, with no time to spend six hours in line and two hours watching. It took a couple of days of increasingly blatant hinting, but eventually I broke through: "Sure! Come down at ten to eight tonight and I'll let you in." Walking past hundreds of folk too surprised to say anything, Judy and I and a couple of friends hustled to the theater and were ushered into the lobby. Once the previous audience left, we were shown into the empty gallery, allowed to choose the best seats in the house. When the Imperial Cruiser passed overhead, all the years of work seemed worth it, even if no more ever came of it than this.

twenty

Commencement Speech

four

Winding down. Starting to feel that I might be ready, I began to hear Vic's music play in my head. Looking for a job. Judy would have loved to have stayed in San Francisco, or to have moved to Puget Sound near her family. But I had a long-term fantasy of coming home to Oregon, owning some acreage, milking horses or whatever those folk do, kicking cowpies with my kid. Being a self-centered surgeon and clueless, we did it my way. I looked for a second car, wanting some cool antique model to drive to work. Sitting in a '49 Cadillac, feeling the familiar cloth on the over-stuffed couch of a seat, the dash with its clicking blinker-arrows, the ivory steering wheel, I remembered my grandfather had had one just like it, me riding in the big back seat when I was five. Sold. (Too elegant, and less than reliable, it sat except for Sunday drives, and I later bought a truck—a mini Japanese pickup, overtly derided by my farmer neighbors.) Not the last of my financial misjudgments, we put our perfect little San Francisco house on the market. If only I'd had the foresight and courage to have kept it and rented it out. . . . But I wanted cash and no burdens to start practice.

Toward the end of each academic year, a party was held for the chief residents, their spouses, and as many other residents as could attend. Junior professors covered the hospitals, and the senior attendings came with their boats. I'd been to a few. The day began with sailing on San Francisco Bay and ended at a yacht club in Marin County. After dinner, one after another, the chiefs would get up and say, "They worked our butts off, it was hard as hell, but this is the best goddamn place in the world and I love you guys." I decided to give a high-school graduation speech. I can't quote it exactly, because I can't find a copy. To get it, you need to know a couple of things: Muriel Steele ran the butt clinic, where we saw lots of venereal warts. And the ileocecal valve is where the small intestine joins the colon, as stool begins the process of changing from unpleasant liquid to manageable solid. I wish I could remember more of the speech, because it was, you'd agree, my finest ever.

"Principal Ebert, faculty, friends, and fellow students of San Francisco High," I began, noting puzzled faces, looking around. "As we gather at this commencement to celebrate an important time in our lives, we must remember those that brought us here. Mr. Blaisdell, our football coach who, when I was hurt, gently said, "RUB IT IN THE DIRT." Miss Steele, our biology teacher, who taught me you don't get warts from frogs. Mr. Trunkey, the ornithologist, who showed me the wonders of the white owl. Mr. Fowler who, when I needed help in chemistry, always said, "huh, huh, huh, eeeehh, huh, huh, huh, eeeehh."

I went on like that for a while, respectfully enumerating the prominent professors—brilliant stuff. Then to the finish: "Commencement means beginning. But this is neither the beginning of life, nor the end. It's the middle of life. More correctly, it's the ileocecal valve of life. For, having come here and worked our way through life's turns and twists and flexures, we are now nearly fully formed, making ready to pass into the glass bowl of reality. Thank you." A standing ovation. I'd hoped Dr. Dunphy would be there; I think he would have liked it.

Afterthoughts

When I left Judy at Travis Air Force Base and headed off to Vietnam, I surprised myself by sobbing like I'd never stop. Three decades later, I'm glad I went. It was the seminal event of my generation; I know it from a perspective held by few of my friends. The analogy to surgical training is imperfect; I chose to be a surgeon, and didn't cry on my way to San Francisco. But it was a tough slog, through a system set up by people over whom I had no control, and with whose conduct within that system I didn't always agree. Nevertheless, I was among the last participants in an era now over for good. I felt part of an unbroken chain of teachers and learners tempered in that same cauldron, walking through the same halls, awake through the same nights, going back for much more than a century. Across the country, the old county hospitals are gone, and the residents are getting a little sleep. I won't argue that it was better then; in fact, it probably wasn't. But my training, which informed the lives of generations of surgeons, in many ways brutal and inhumane, is an experience I feel privileged to have had before it disappeared forever.

I wonder if Dr. Dunphy and his WW II buddies, and those before them, actually had thought it out like this, as they fashioned the modern rules of training surgeons: beat them down, overwork them, hold back the rewards, so that only those who really love it, who find being a surgeon irresistible—like surrendering to a disease—will push on into the senior years of residency. If people burn up and drop out, good riddance. Take their mistakes and wave them like semaphores, visible for miles. There are no brighter lights than those in an operating room. You'd better get used to it, because there's no separating from the pleasure of dramatic success the misery of abject failure. Fear of failure is the surgeon's safety net, and his dead weight. If you haven't had driven into your essence the sweaty recognition that failure is just around the corner, you ought never pick up a knife. But if you aren't the kind to overlook that fear and plow ahead believing you're prepared, you'll never get out of bed in the morning, much less in the middle of the night.

For me, it was a marriage made in limbo. I think I got pretty good at it; I was listed in a national guide to America's top doctors (sounds better than it is), and I got highly favorable annual patient survey results (that meant something). Until the data were quashed by protests from other doctors, the biggest local insurance company gave out certain yearly statistics. My costs per case, my hospital days per operation were among the very lowest in the state. Doctors and nurses wanted me to care for them; ninety-nine percent of my patients did fine. None of that satisfied me. The one percent drove me crazy with second-guessing and self-recrimination. I lay awake at night, and got to hate the telephone. I missed a lot of family events. Where's the balance? When is it ok to look at an imperfect outcome and say you did your best, instead of filling yourself with remorse and self-doubt? Is time off a betrayal of trust? Can you ever get over a mistake? Should you? Where does confidence end and delusion begin? Once you open a person up, do you ever close?

And it's worse now than it ever was. When I first went into practice in Oregon, my partners asked me how many operations a week I thought I'd want to do. I hadn't thought about it. Ten? You'll kill yourself, they said. Six is perfect. You'll feel useful, you'll make a good enough living, and you'll have some time to enjoy life. Twenty years later, I was often doing more than twenty cases a week. (Vic did his eighteen, but he didn't take emergency calls, and had house staff to do lots of the work.) Continuously falling reimbursement had much to do with it. More perverse: unlike a lawyer, an artist, or nearly any other professional, what you get has nothing to do with the quality of your work. Here's what we pay for a colon resection, says Medicare, say the millionaire insurance execs. We don't care if your patients do better or if your costs are lower than anyone else. And we sure as hell don't care if your anastomoses are *artful* (making sarcastic quotation marks in the air, with their inky fingers), whatever the hell that means. And don't even start on that *music* bullshit.

Looking back on those times in San Francisco, mostly with pride and amazement that I did it, it's impossible not to consider the present state of medical care in America and worry. And I do: about the care, and the care-givers. We should, as Don Trunkey used to say (he used to say lots of things, as you now know), keep our eyes on the doughnut and not the hole. In American health care we are, in fact, looking deeply into the hole. Everyone knows it costs too much and it's unevenly distributed—absent altogether for lots of folks. The best medical care in the world is available in the US. Right there next to some of the worst. Is it fixable? I think it comes down to three perfectly simple questions: 1) How much do we want to pay for health care? 2) How can we best control costs? 3) What kind of people do we want taking care of us?

The first question is, in theory, the easiest. All we need to do as a society is calculate how much we can afford and want to spend on health care. Which means all we need to do is elect politicians who care about solutions, and are willing to seek them regardless of party politics. That will happen tomorrow, right? And, having done that, and figured out how big the pot is, we simply decide which kinds of medical care deserve what sort of priorities. It's just math, and realism. Simple. So while you're getting out your slide rule, I'll move on to the second question, because it's in fact related to the first.

So far there's only been one approach to cost control (packaged in various disguises): cut payments to doctors and hospitals. But there's only so much blood in that particular turnip; and there comes a point at which the purpose is defeated. We're well past that point: hospitals are in trouble all over the country, doctors and nurses are burning out nearly as fast as they're being produced, and care is no more available than it ever was. The time is long overdue to focus—while we avoid the elephant on the sofa known as rationing—on figuring out what sorts of care make the most economic sense. Here's my favorite example, which, of course, applies directly to me and makes me look brilliant: those gallbladder operations I've described from my training era are long gone. We made large incisions, and patients routinely stayed in the hospital for up to a week. Now, laparoscopic surgery (making about four small incisions and inserting a camera and long thin tools, while watching what we do on a video screen) has replaced that, and patients are typically going home the same day as their operation. That's a good thing. But before laparoscopic surgery came about, I'd worked on getting gallbladders out through smaller and smaller incisions, with shorter and shorter stays; eventually getting down to one or one-and-a-half inches and same-day discharge. What's the difference? Two or three thousand dollars per case in cost: those scopes and fancy tools are expensive. Others found the same thing. Studies have been done showing no difference between "mini" gallbladder surgery and laparoscopic surgery in terms of postop pain, recovery time, and back-to-work time, and have confirmed the cost difference. But virtually no one is doing mini gallbladder surgery. Why? Because, among other things, laparoscopic surgery has been hyped and advertised, and there's a huge amont of money behind it, so it's what people think they want. (And it's easier to do!)

Likewise, surgeons are now doing all sorts of other operations laparoscopically. Colon surgery is a good example. Again, claims

I love this: when I took my first laparoscopy course, it was all about lasers. In fact, the gallbladder operation was called "LLC," for laser laparoscopic cholecystectomy. Laser companies sponsored the courses and tried to get everyone to buy their product, for tens of thousands of dollars. But we also learned with old-fashioned electrocautery. Seeing no advantage for the laser, I asked the rep, why buy one? "Because," he said, "it's what people want. If they hear you're doing it without a laser, they'll go elsewhere." Which, for a while, was true. (I've been asked hundreds of times, regarding nearly any operation, if it could be done with a laser— as if it were some sort of miracle tool.) I can testify that there are lots of laser machines gathering dust outside operating rooms. I once read an article in a surgical journal that trumpeted: since we've been using a laser for mastectomy, our blood transfusion level has gone from four to two units, and hospitalization from six to four days. My god! I (and nearly every surgeon I knew) never needed to give blood for a mastectomy, and I saw people home in one or two days.

are made of more rapid recovery and shorter hospital times. People go home in three to five days, instead of a week or longer. The operations take more time, and the operating room costs are higher, but because of quicker discharge, there are overall savings. But wait: a few of us old-fart surgeons can remove colons through relatively small incisions, taking a quarter of the operating time, requiring none of the use-once-and-throw-away laparoscopic equipment (which piles up in landfills), and seeing the patients go home happy and comfortable in two or three days, saving thousands of dollars. But there's no mechanism for encouraging such choice-making, and that applies to non-surgical care as well.

Some doctors, for reasons including skill and willingness to work their rear-ends off, produce better results than other doctors. Yet efforts are just beginning to identify them, to figure out what they are doing that others aren't, and to spread the word. Not to mention rewarding those doctors. And here's the essence of the perversity, which, coincidentally, gets to the third point as well: we're in the process, subtly but meaningfully, of selecting an entirely different sort of person who chooses health-care as a profession. There will always be people for whom medicine is a calling and a committment, to whom no amount of frustration will be enough to deter them from giving good care. But the system is increasingly stacked against attracting and keeping such folk. For better or worse, the kind of training I experienced was a fine filter: you can't go into and through something like that without a real commitment to the profession. It's easier to become a doctor now (as fewer people choose to, medical schools are having to lower standards) but it's becoming much less fulfilling, as the core satisfactions are overwhelmed by bullshit.

In all my years of medical school and surgical training, I never once heard anyone say they were in it for the money. Yet I think there's been an implicit understanding—as there ought to be— that hard work and the production of excellence will in some way be commensurately rewarded. Isn't that what we all want of our lives? Most of us make major life-choices with inadequate information. (I stumbled into a great marriage for all the wrong reasons, for example.) But the word is getting out: the profession of medicine is less and less about quality and more and more about the bottom line. Take a look at the business office of a large clinic or hospital: there dozens and dozens of people in cubicles doing nothing but insurance paperwork. Multiply that by thousands of health insurance companies across the country, sucking up billions of healthcare dollars (and distributing lots of it in executive salaries and investor profits). Doctors—even the ones with deep commitment—are helpless against the tide of paperwork, the demands and restrictions of insurance companies, the increasing overhead. If you don't give cash flow a high priority, you will get washed away. It's hard not to become exactly what you never wanted to be: a money-grubbing automaton. I'll agree that many doctors used to make way too much money. But times have changed.

So who will choose medicine if it's true that those who pay for it—insurance companies and government—continue to make no distinction between those who provide a higher-quality product and those who don't? People who believe in excellence will look elsewhere for professional satisfaction. Trust me: it's happening. Exactly the sort of people you'd like to become your doctor are choosing not to. When, during training, I expressed concern about my future in a crowded profession, Dr. Dunphy

Cutting Remarks

said, "There's always room at the top." I went through a system that demanded much, but which also held out a promise. I'm not so sure anymore.

Some people say you have to be brave to be a surgeon. Vic Richards said, "The patient takes all the risk, Dockie." What is it, exactly, that gives one human being the right to stick a hand deep into another's most squishy essence and feel around? I haven't figured it out. But I know there was nothing else I could have been. I was born for it. And at least I could tell when I was finished with an operation. As opposed to writing a goddamn book.

About the Author

SIDNEY M. SCHWAB, MD, Board Certified in Surgery and a Fellow of the American College of Surgeons, did his surgery training at the University of California at San Francisco and practiced surgery in Oregon and Washington State, where he served on the board of directors of one of the most successful fully physician-run multispecialty clinics in the U.S. Schwab has been listed in a national guide to top doctors. Today he lives in Everett, Washington, with Judy Mumma Schwab, his wife of thirty-four years.